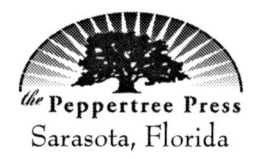

Reprise

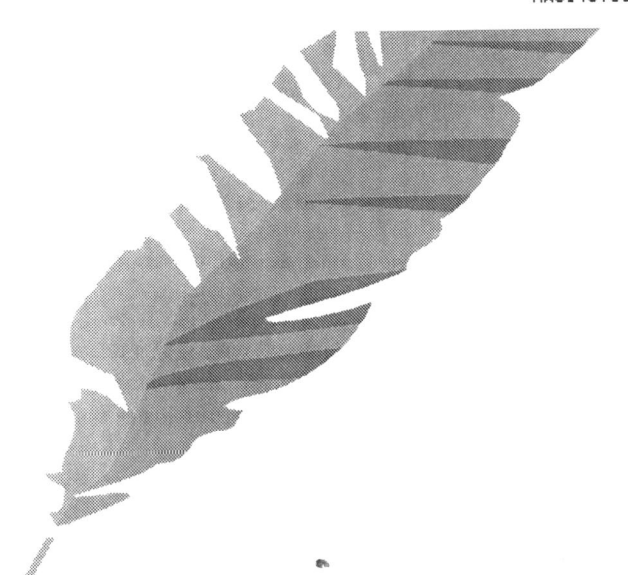

by Rich Brooks

the Peppertree Press
Sarasota, Florida

Copyright © Rich Brooks, 2007

All rights reserved. Published by the Peppertree Press, LLC.

the Peppertree Press and associated logos are trademarks of the Peppertree Press, LLC.

No part of this publication may be reproduced, stored in a retrieval system, transmitted in any form or by any means, electronic, mechanical, photocopying, recording, or otherwise, without prior written permission of the publisher and author/illustrator.

Graphic design by Rebecca Warrick Barbier

Cover by Roger Skelton

For information regarding permissions, write to
the Peppertree Press, LLC.,
Attention: Publisher,
1269 First Street, Suite 7
Sarasota, Florida 34236

ISBN:9781934246-88-7

Library of Congress Number: 2007942046

Printed in the U.S.A.

Printed December 2007

Rich Brooks' columns appear in the Sarasota Herald-Tribune and are reprinted with the permission of the Herald-Tribune media group.

Introduction

The dictionary defines reprise as a "repetition of a song or part of a song... To take again."

And that's what this book is. A reprise of the columns I've written since 1997, roughly two years after I was diagnosed with ALS, or Lou Gehrig's disease.

I started writing the columns as a way to continue contributing to the daily newspaper, a business that I've been affiliated with since carrying the Citizen-Journal as a boy growing up in Columbus, Ohio.

More than words though, these columns are a chronicle of a life with ALS.

There's the column I wrote in 1997 in which I first told readers that I have ALS

And there's the column I wrote, also in 1997, lamenting the things I can no longer do.

I also tackle some controversial topics, such as potty training, visits from relatives and cutting the lawn. In another way, the columns also chronicle my encounters with technology designed to help me write.

In the ten years I've written this column I've gone from typing, to using voice recognition software to dictating it to a health aid. I now use a laptop computer equipped with text to voice software that speaks for me. It also has an infrared switch that allows me to write.

Not surprisingly, many columns deal with family life and struggling to adapt to a degenerative and often terminal disease.

What does a war correspondent write about? About the topic that consumes him and is part of his being. I also write about the topics that consume me. Think of me as a correspondent writing from the front of life.

Rich Brooks
November 2007

Forward

When Rich Brooks joined the newsroom staff of the Sarasota Herald-Tribune more than 20 years ago, he was feisty and opinionated, with a stiletto witthat never cut too close to the jugular. His dead-pan sarcasm was the perfect foil for a tender heart. I would describe him the same way today. What has changed is purely physical. Until 1995, when he was diagnosed with amyotrophic lateral sclerosis – Lou Gehrig's disease – he could throw the football with his sons, play a respectable round of golf with his buddies, leap from his La-Z-Boy when the Buckeyes scored a touchdown, and wrap his arms around Kathy, his wife of 29 years. Now he is confined to a wheelchair, hooked up to a ventilator and a feeding tube, virtually motionless and unable to speak. A disease as mean as Lou Gehrig's can either scare its victim into submission or provoke a fight. Rich Brooks put up his dukes and has never stopped fighting. He's still feisty and opinionated. Still funny. And, beneath that matter-of-fact air, still tender. Eleven years after his diagnosis, Rich continues to write his award-winning column for the Herald-Tribune. He uses a laptop computer with an infrared switch to scan the alphabet. It is a laborious process, but you would never know it by reading his confident prose. He deals with all sorts of topics, recounting life events as simple as getting a 14-year-old to mow the lawn and as profound as choosing a ventilator over certain death. What resonates most with readers is his grasp of what's important in life: family, friends, community. Rich has lived with ALS well past the five-year prognosis that comes with this unfathomable diagnosis. Those who know him fully expect that he will persevere for many years more. That's as much a tribute to Kathy and their sons, Noah and Nathaniel, as it is to Rich's strength and sense of purpose. Rich finds fulfillment in his work. He says his readers have helped keep him alive. He, in turn, has challenged us to live our lives to the fullest!

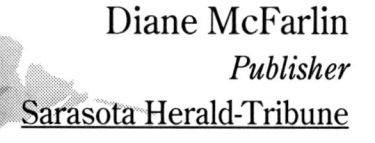

Diane McFarlin
Publisher
Sarasota Herald-Tribune

Table of Contents

April 12, 1997
    Despite frailties, we reach for the stars   1

May 25, 1997
    Uncle Bobby, the pilot I never met   3

May 31, 1997
    All I want for class is my lost tooth   5

July 19, 1997
    No more hand-cranked hash   7

July 26, 1997
    Friends, neighbors help those in need   9

Sepember 26.1997
    So much I would, if only I could   11

May 30, 1998
    Mornings devoted to walk and roll   13

June 6, 1998
    Kids, guns pose hard questions, decisions   15

October 24, 1998
    Lottery winner, give me a call   17

February 20, 1999
    My Mother enters the computer age   19

February 27, 1999
    Dad's crooked pitch misses the plate   21

April 24, 1999
    Mundane moments can't be all that bad   23

June 19, 1999
    Remembering dad: the good and the bad   25

July 17, 1999
    4 birds in the cage worth 3 in the snake   27

October 2 1999
    The mark of a proud but annoying parent   29

October 30, 1999
   The great dilemma of trick-or-treating 31

December 18, 1999
   How times change: joys of chopping 33

January 15, 2000
   Frustration grew as the minutes ticked away 35

January 22, 2000
   Humor is good for the heart, soul 37

March 18, 2000
   It's a home invasion 39

April 22, 2000
   Wheelchairs crimp restaurant dining 41

July 22, 2000
   Family games illuminates competition 43

August 5, 2000
   Exploring the different meanings of growth 45

September 25, 2000
   Slipping in and out of the digital age 47

December 30, 2000
   Remembering the reasons for the holidays 49

May 5, 2001
   Reaching a state of denial 51

May 12, 2001
   Mother's day: who loves ya, baby? 53

August 18, 2001
   Parenthood and the power to annoy 55

November 17, 2001
   Following the path of Lou Gehrig 57

October 19, 2002
   A family that works together is better able to
   work things out together 59

January 11, 2003
    Forray into parochial school proves scary   61

March 1, 2003
    Lion and saint: saying goodbye to Two-Drink Betty   63

May 24, 2003
    Facing untimely demise, boyhood has unlikely savior   65

August 9, 2003
    To the hosipatal staff: it's been great,
    but I don't want to see you again   67

August 16, 2003
    Struggle for home ventilator is a fight for like   69

September 20, 2003
    Mid-term's cosmic report card   71

November 22, 2003
    No matter how much is taken away,
    you always have something left   73

February 28, 2004
    Like this artist's renderings,
    life doesn't always paint inside the lines   75

April 24, 2004
    Buttering corn on the cob and living life
    can both offer challenges   79

May 1, 2004
    North Port Commission could learn something
    from Pope Stephen VII   81

September 11, 2004
    Small talk becomes a big thing
    when you're no longer able to do it   83

October 16, 2004
    Sign of the times: temperature drops,
    but air conditioner keeps running   85

November 20, 2004
   Giving thanks: mending fences, good neighbors
   and Harley Davidson   87

February 5, 2005
   State of parenthood: suffering from delusions   89

March 19, 2005
   Warning: teen brain under construction
   may cause cleaning frenzy   91

May 7, 2005
   For fun or profit, mowing the lawn has its own reward   93

August 6, 2005
   Aliens among us?
   Back-to-school shopping provides close encounter   95

September 3, 2005
   Praise for teen surprises parents   97

November 19, 2005
   Goodbye turkey: it's been great   99

December 10, 2005
   Christmas definetely a work in progress   101

June 24, 2006
   Refugees teach us valuable lesson   103

December 23, 2006
   Your kindness was not unnoticed   105

January 27, 2007
   It's good to be the bad guy, sometimes   107

May 26, 2007
   Embrace mortality, then live and grow   109

July 14, 2007
   The trendy side of proactive parenting   111

July 28, 2007
   A friend's acceptance of death is hard to take   113

April 12, 1997

Despite frailties, we reach for stars

We shuffled along the walkway, each of us clinging to a guide rope. A chuck-will's-widow called out from across a patch of moolli grass, scrub and sand dunes. Overhead, the stars seemed to burst out in a glow. The Hale-Bopp comet appeared ghostlike in the northwestern sky.

A good night for star gazing. A good night for the New Moon Party on Tuesday at Shamrock Park in South Venice.

With park supervisor Nial Pace leading, we walked silently along the nature trail toward the Intracoastal Waterway, letting the sights, sounds and smells of the warm spring evening fill our senses.

I let go of the rope.

"Are we going too fast for you?" volunteer Bessie Kofsky asked as the group forged ahead.

"I'll manage," I grunted and hobbled along. Something wasn't right. My left leg was being less cooperative than usual, and I struggled to maintain my footing like a drunken sailor on deck in a storm. Maybe it was fatigue.

I thought about my cane, and regretted leaving it in my van. My ego wouldn't let me bring it along. I didn't want anyone to think I needed a cane.

We reached an access road. The group crossed. I didn't. Two, maybe three steps later, my left foot caught on the pebbled asphalt.

"Oh —!," I groaned as I spilled onto the pavement.

"Are you all right?" Mrs. Kofsky asked.

On my hands and knees, I crawled to a nearby wooden pylon, hugged it and resurrected myself.

"Everything OK back there?" Nial called from the front of the formation.

"I'm OK," I said to Mrs. Kofsky. "Nothing hurt but my pride."

Crossing the road, Mrs. Kofsky was clearly worried about my abilities. She illuminated the path before me with a flashlight. Dodging stubby palmettos and tree stumps, we snaked our way down a narrow trail, the toe of the Nike on my left foot occasionally dragging in the dirt.

I tumbled again, this time landing in the soft sand.

Mrs. Kofsky grabbed my shoulder and tried to right me, but she was not strong enough. Allan Sacharow, a park staff member, stooped and looped his arm around my shoulders, hoisting me to my feet.

He let go reluctantly, not sure I could maintain my balance.

After a brief exchange with Nial, Allan left to retrieve a park vehicle to take me back to my van. Mrs. Kofsky waited with me, and the group moved onward.

Gazing at the night sky, I thought back to more than a year ago.

My wife, Kathy, and I were sitting in a neurologist's office, waiting for him to tell me why I couldn't hit a drive any farther than 180 yards; why I couldn't lift a 40-pound bag of salt; why, when I walked, I felt as if I had swim fins on my feet.

"Are you saying he has ALS?" she asked. She squeezed my hand, and I saw tears welling up in her hazel eyes.

Amiotrophic lateral sclerosis - killer of the great Lou Gehrig.

The words sank in. I felt as a mastadon might have felt struggling in a tar pit, raging against an enemy that can't be fought.

"That's Jupiter," Mrs. Kofsky said, pointing overhead to the brightest light in the sky.

Arriving home, I was sullen. Angry I didn't gather enough material for a column. Embarrassed I made such a spectacle of myself. Good thing it was dark.

Kathy, who seems to be at her best when I am at my worst, chided me.

"Stop hiding your disability," she said.

To the back porch I walked, and found myself looking skyward. Clouds had moved in, and the comet had drifted below the horizon.

I thought of Alan Shepherd, John Glenn, Neil Armstrong - humanity's yearning to reach for the stars while dealing with our frailties.

Then the irony hit me.

That's me, a metaphor for humanity: reaching for the stars while falling on my butt.

May 25, 1997

Uncle Bobby, the pilot I never met

Uncle Bobby is standing next to a fighter plane. His left arm resting on the wing, his left foot on the tire.

Above his head are the grinning teeth of a tiger, or perhaps a shark, painted on the plane's engine cover. A painted eye behind the propeller stares menacingly at the camera.

There's no text or date on the 2½ - inch - square picture. I'm guessing that the plane is an early version of the Mustang, and, judging from the barren landscape, that the airfield is in North Africa, where Uncle Bobby was stationed in 1942.

Uncle Bobby is dressed in his tropical uniform, which included shorts, knee-high socks and a short-sleeve shirt. On his chest are the wings of a Flight Officer of the Royal Canadian Air Force.

I never met Uncle Bobby. He was killed before I was born. On a foggy day, April 22, 1943, Flight Officer Robert Burns Reed crashed his Mustang while landing at an airfield near Sussex, England. The crash investigation listed "poor visibility" as the cause.

He had been transferred to the base only about a week before. My Mom, Bobby's sister, said there was some speculation that Uncle Bobby was not familiar with the airfield and overshot the landing strip.

Nevertheless, I have come to know Uncle Bobby through the letters he wrote to his home in Lowellville, Ohio - a village outside Youngstown fed by the steel mills of the Mahoning River Valley. I also have pictures, his RCAF flight log and other correspondence.

Uncle Bobby was attending Ole Miss in 1940. When he was a senior, barely old enough to legally drink liquor, he quit school and joined up with the RCAF.

His letters - words sculpted in crisp slashes and loops on stationery so thin that it is nearly transparent - tell of hot days and cool nights in an

Egyptian desert, Messerschmitts' machine guns stabbing at supply convoys and bases, and bouts with tedium and boredom.

From a base outside Alexandria, he wrote to my parents, congratulating them on the birth of their first child, my older sister:

"I'm not in a particularly jocular mood today - we just finished burying four men, our men, who were killed yesterday in a bombing raid . . . I thought it was Junkers 88 by the sound of its motor - I was flat on my face in a trench and didn't get to see it."

In another letter, he wrote of being "disgusted" at having to retreat as Erwin Rommel's Afrika Corps advanced.

"I'd rather stay and fight . . . but headquarters says move," he wrote.

Reading Uncle Bobby's letters made me wonder what life would have been like if he had not been killed in the war.

I would have grown up listening to Uncle Bobby's fighter pilot stories.

He would have been the hit at Easter family reunions at Aunt Margaret's in Kent, Ohio, dazzling us with tales of strafing enemy fortifications or streaking over treetops, photographing German positions in western France.

With his pilot's training, he would have been plucked by a commercial airline after the war and married his Lowellville High sweetheart.

Later, with grandchildren swirling about, he would retire to a bungalow on Casey Key. I would have him over for cookouts on weekends, and he would dazzle my sons with tales of his adventures as an RCAF fighter pilot.

We would play golf with my Mom; I would give him 3-foot putts and buy him gin and tonics in the clubhouse.

My grandmother was at Good Friday services when, in 1943, she got word of Uncle Bobby's death. A priest at Holy Rosary, a small Roman Catholic church on Wood Street in Lowellville, told her as she was walking through the huge oak doors at the rear of the church. My grandfather had dispatched a messenger to the church with the urgent telegram.

A simple white wooden cross in the Canadian ground at Brookwood Cemetery in Surrey, England, marks Uncle Bobby's grave. He was 24 when he died.

Monday, I plan to celebrate Memorial Day by taking my sons to the beach. And every time a plane flies overhead, I will think of Uncle Bobby, the life he had, and the life he didn't have.

May 31, 1997

All I want for class is my lost tooth

Up and down, back and forth the 6-year-old wiggled the tooth, his eyes alternately rolling and squinting in syncopated rhythm.

"Is it bleeding?" he asked my wife as she read to him a Dr. Seuss story.

"Just a little," was the reply.

Finally, the tooth popped out.

"Look, Dad," he said with a snaggletoothed grin while proudly displaying the enamel prize in the palm of his hand.

Instead of cashing in the tooth with the Tooth Fairy, though, the 6-year-old had other plans. Losing the tooth gave him a membership to the exclusive Open Space Club in his kindergarten class. And to make sure the TF did not abscond with the loot, he carefully hid the tooth under a book on his night stand.

"See?" he said, revealing the hiding place. "She will look under my pillow, but it won't be there."

"He won't find it," he added, apparently unsure if the TF is male or female.

The following day, the 6-year-old was relieved to find the tooth was where he left it. And there was no sign that the TF had rifled his room in a search for the booty.

So after breakfast, he packed up the tooth for transport to school. First he placed it in a fresh paper cup, which was then covered with aluminum foil. Then the cup, foil and tooth were secured in a plastic sandwich bag with a sealed top.

He was taking no chances. He wanted to make sure his teacher could verify that he had, indeed, lost one of his front teeth, as if the gaping hole in his smile was not evidence enough.

To get into the club, according to teacher Laura Simanskey, the student has to lose a tooth and then tell the class how the deed was done. There are no other rights and privileges involved.

But to kindergarteners, belonging is everything.

They know that losing baby teeth is part of growing up, which they are anxious to do. They wear their toothless grins as if they were medals indicating that they are becoming Big Kids.

"They've all been pulling on their teeth since January," Mrs. Simanskey said. "I have to remind them to keep their fingers out of their mouths because of the germs."

Parents watch these passages - first communions, graduations, marriage - with mixed emotions. They are proud that the offspring are thriving, yet wishing to somehow slow the march of time and preserve their kids in preschool innocence.

And yet, as my own mother reminds me, healthy birds fly away.

Firmly initiated into the Open Spaces Club, the 6-year-old put the tooth on his night stand the following night and found a buck in its place in the morning, placed it in his bank and will soon forget about it.

But he will always be a member of the Open Spaces Club. Some things are more important than money. Just about every 6-year-old knows that.

Speaking of teeth . . .

The Venice Area Chamber of Commerce is looking for a few good teeth.

No, we're not talking about the choppers you keep in a glass by your bed.

We're talking fossils here.

The chamber is seeking folks who collect fossils and sharks teeth. Collectors are needed for the Sixth Annual Sharks Tooth & Seafood Festival coming up in August.

Only serious collectors need apply.

"We're looking for people who have substantial collections of fossilized sharks teeth and dinosaur bones," said Charlie Cronk, chamber spokesman.

In other words, they don't want folks who sift through the sand at Caspersen Beach and plop their findings into an empty mayonaise jar at home.

Cronk said there are a few openings in the festival's fossil tent for aficionados to display and sell their collections.

The festival includes arts and crafts, music and food. But the fossil tent is the heart of the festival for the city that bills itself "Sharks Tooth Capital of the World."

Anyone interested can call Cronk at 488-2236. He'll fill you in on the details.

July 19, 1997

No more hand-cranked hash

The wave is dead. As is the mouse.

So, our household has plunged into a technological stone age - into a time before noodles were called pasta and only rich people had telephones in their cars.

We aren't exactly living in a cave and spearing wild hogs for dinner. But the loss two months ago of the microwave (something blew up inside) and the computer mouse last week (a problem with the component that runs the mouse), is forcing us to make some adjustments.

Folks at our house are far from being techno wizards, or whatever the clever catch phrase is these days for those on the cutting edge of home computers and technology.

We judge technology not by the amount of gigabytes or size of RAM, but by its usefulness to our everyday lives.

During the school year, the 11-year-old used the computer for book reports, science papers and other forays into academia. Of course, this was after he was flogged for waiting until the last minute to start writing.

The 6-year-old likes to play educational games, which seem to help him with shapes, letters and patterns.

For me, the computer helps keep track of the family finances and checking account. I also use it for letters and notes for this column. We also occasionally get e-mail from our cousins up north.

Life without the computer has been inconvenient, at worst.

More significant has been the loss of the microwave.

The microwave, rest its beeping soul, made meal preparation quick and convenient.

For families where both parents work (that's us) this is nothing to sniff at. Leftover macaroni and cheese, enchiladas, hot dogs and other epicurean delights could be popped in to the wave for a minute or so, and presto, a meal fit for a 6-year-old.

Without it, remnants of family meals languish in the fridge, usually until a brave soul peels back the foil cover, sniffs the contents and exclaims, "Eeewwww! What's this?"

We've tried to adjust, with mixed results.

A couple of weeks ago, I used some leftover corned beef to make hash. I won't bore you with the recipe, but I pulled it out of a cookbook written before cholesterol became a household watchword.

I even ad libbed - that's what hash is all about - substituting experienced Tater Tots for "cooked chopped potatoes' called for in the recipe.

I had purchased a hand-crank meat grinder at a garage sale a couple of years ago, so my 6-year-old and one of the neighborhood kids ground the meat and tots into a pulpy pink mixture.

The result, probably because it was cooked in oil and the corned beef was loaded with fat to begin with, was greasy hash.

We ending up pitching the concoction, opting for fast-food burgers.

Technology has a price, and it's lightening my wallet.

Higher food bills. Kaa-ching!

One-hundred-fifty pops for a new computer motherboard. Kaa-ching!

Four hundred bucks for a new over-the-stove microwave. Kaa-ching!

So this weekend, I'll be shopping for a new microwave and surfing the net for a Luddite home page.

Technology is a semi-wonderful thing.

July 26, 1997

Friends, neighbors help those in need

Pulling into the driveway, I noticed it immediately.

The lawn was cut, trimmed and edged.

I'd left my mom's house, north of Orlando, just after lunch Monday, figuring to arrive home by midafternoon to cut the lawn before settling into my easy chair for happy hour.

But the Yard Fairies beat me to it.

The Yard Fairies, neighbors Kyle, John and Rick, have made quite a few visits to our homestead.

A couple of months ago, Kyle installed an underground sprinkling system in our front yard. A few weeks later, he and John joined a family effort to lay two pallets of sod.

And where my yard once resembled a strip-mining operation, or a dirt playground for dogs and armadillos, there is now a lush lawn.

After that, I found my lawnmower had broken down, so I borrowed Rick's brand new Sears riding mower to cut my lawn. While I swept up and down the sloping front yard, Rick used a weed-wacker to trim the grass in the culverts, around the fence and swing set - anywhere the twin 42-inch blades with mulching action couldn't reach.

The following week, Kyle and I (90 percent Kyle) repaired the gas line on my aging riding lawnmower. After the required six trips to the hardware store for parts, we found that it was the battery that had died.

So Kyle scooted around on his mower while I watched.

"Thanks," I said after the last stand of grass fell to the blade of John Deere.

"No problem," he said as he puttered into the fading sunlight like a suburban Lone Ranger.

There are lots of folks, such as myself, with various forms of physical disabilities who find themselves on the receiving end of such generosities.

But there are also those who need help but are too proud to ask, and those who want to help but are afraid, or don't know how, to offer.

Depression, anger and frustration are what victims of stroke, Parkinson's disease, and other afflictions feel when they find they can no longer do the chores and activities they did when they were healthy.

"They feel like they are no longer contributing members of the family," said Dr. Cynthia Bailey, director of psychology at HealthSouth of Sarasota, a rehabilitation facility.

Independence and self-sufficiency are the foundations of pride and self-esteem.

Accomplishing tasks that most of us take for granted - laundry, cleaning house, pulling weeds, driving a car - can be daunting or impossible for those who, after a lifetime of work, homemaking or child-rearing, find themselves with weakened or useless limbs.

"Many people get depressed and frustrated when they find that they won't get any better," Dr. Bailey said. For them, it's better to "look for other ways to contribute, rather than dwell on what they can no longer accomplish.

"Neighbors and friends are often acutely aware of what's going on. Sometimes, the problem is that the person needing help won't ask for it. Or the friends don't know what to do or say . . . They just need to ask, 'What can I do?' or just cut the lawn or whatever."

For many disabled people, getting around is the hardest part. Bailey suggested that a simple way to get involved is to offer a ride.

"People can feel trapped in their houses. They have no way to get to the store or doctor. Offering to drive them somewhere may not seem like much, but it can be a big help," she said.

I'm sure there are lots of other folks out there who, like The Yard Fairies, pitch in and help. Their reward may come in the form of a neighborhood cookout, a beer, a batch of home-baked sugar cookies, or just a "Thank you" and a smile.

September 26, 1997

So much I would, if only I could

If I could, I would shed these splints on my legs and run again.

Springing out of bed, I would jog for two miles every morning - well, maybe just three days a week - and when I got back, I would pack school lunches and pour bowls of Cheerios before the boys rubbed the sleep from their eyes.

I would not need help to get dressed, and I would iron my own shirts, just as I used to.

My first thoughts of the day would have nothing to do with the awful truth of this Lou Gehrig's disease, diagnosed two years ago. It's a disease that leaves my hands too weak to grip, my shoulders and arms atrophied, and my legs fighting for balance even when I'm standing still.

If I could, I would show my sons, Noah and Nathaniel, how to shoot a jumper by raising the ball high above their heads and not releasing it until their feet reached their peak. I would show them how to make free throws and layups, and no-look passes to a forward breaking to the basket.

We would play Horse, Pig and Around the World. I'm sure our neighbors wouldn't mind if we used their court.

On Sunday mornings, I would get up early and make a huge breakfast - the kind my dad used to make. We would pig out on sausage gravy, eggs and sliced tomatoes grown in our back yard.

After breakfast, we would go to church. Walking down the aisle, my gait would be steady and proud, not the limping hobble that tasks me now. My wife, Kathy, would lead, and my sons would each take one of my hands.

After church, the boys and I would go to the beach, giving Kathy some time to herself. I would hoist 6-year-old Nathaniel up on my shoulders while Noah, wearing a dive mask, would grab my legs under water. Then we would fall backward into the warm Gulf, spitting salt water and sand when we came up.

The waves wouldn't knock me down, and I wouldn't need help to navigate my way back to our chairs and towels.

If I could, I would help my wife with the laundry. I would mop the floors and clean the bathrooms, just as I used to.

On Saturday afternoons, we would go for a bike ride and buy ice cream cones at the citrus stand. Orange for me, chocolate for Nathaniel, vanilla for Noah; and Kathy would get an orange-vanilla swirl.

The ice cream would run down the sides of the cones, and we would all have sticky hands and fingers.

On Saturday nights, maybe once a month, Kathy and I would go ballroom dancing. We would waltz, cha-cha, rhumba and fox trot to intoxicating rhythms. Sometimes, I would step on her toes, or she would step on mine, and we would kiss after each dance.

On my hands and knees, I would crawl through our butterfly garden, pulling each weed out by its roots, then throwing it on the grass to shrivel in the sun.

My fingernails would get black from the dirt, and I would scrub them clean with an old toothbrush saved for that purpose.

We would play golf as a family - Kathy would object, but would go along to be a good sport - and I would show the boys how to play sand shots.

In the fall, we would fly to Columbus for a long weekend and go to an Ohio State football game. We would climb the dozen or so flights of stadium stairs and sit in the sun on C-deck, where we would dine on hot dogs and Cokes.

The family room and living room need painting, and I would do that, no longer worried about dropping a wet brush on the rug or falling off a ladder. With steady hands, I would repair the screen door on the back porch.

On some evenings, I would fetch my guitar and plunk out a Neil Young tune, or maybe teach the boys three-part harmony so we could sing "Tom Dooley."

And each night, I would thank the Creator for this grand life and health, instead of asking, "Why me?"

But I give thanks for my life, anyway.

May 30, 1998

Mornings devoted to walk and roll

It had been a few days since we were able to take our morning walk together.

And as Friday morning revealed itself warm and humid, but lacking the drizzling rain of the two previous days, the 7-year-old was anxious to return to our routine.

As soon as he chomped down the last of his peanut butter-and-jelly on toast breakfast, he was knocking on the bedroom door as my wife and I struggled with my socks, shoes and leg splints.

In families with two working parents, as well as single-parent households, school mornings can be hectic times. Kids need to be dressed, fed, backpacks checked, hair combed, teeth brushed, lunches packed.

The family slaves (parents) need to shower, dress and get ready for a day at the salt mines.

After my wife and the 12-year-old hit the road, the 7-year-old (a.k.a No. 2 Son) and I have 20 minutes or so for our walk.

It's not a walk, really, as much as a roll: me in my motorized wheelchair, No. 2 Son in his rollerblades. Sometimes we are accompanied by the whippet, who at 11 years old can still outrun anything with four legs in the neighborhood.

There are only a half dozen streets and 30 or so homes in our neck of the woods, so our morning route varies only slightly.

On Friday our path turned right at the bottom of the driveway. No. 2 Son falls in behind and latches on to the wheelchair, allowing me to pull him along as if he were on water skis.

"Do we have time for a long walk, today?" he asks as he glides past.

"Sure do," I say.

We pass his girlfriend's house, then a vacant lot dotted with wild grasses that have tiny star-shaped flowers. The whippet sniffs at them suspiciously and prances on.

Another turn and we come upon a fenced yard where four miniature schnauzers roam. One has recently produced a litter of pups, says the 7-year-old.

But the pups are not out, and the dogs bark their warning at our approach.

We roll on and talk.

He tells me that a friend's father once shot an alligator twice in the head and the gator lived. This happened in a cave. "And the cave was hot. Whew!"

This leads to a conversation about what alligators eat.

"Fish and feet," I say.

"Daaaad! You're jokin'," says he.

Then I pose a question sure to embarrass him.

"Ever smooch your girlfriend?"

"No," is his flat reply.

The talk turns to school.

Art, he tells me, is his favorite subject.

This is not a surprise, considering that he has shown some talent in that area and is encouraged by a good teacher whose classroom he says is "real messy."

We pass the home of his friend Kenny and round the final bend.

Ahead we see a mockingbird dive-bombing the whippet, which leaps and nearly snaps the aerial attacker from the sky.

At home we make the final rounds through the house, gathering his lunch and backpack. As we scurry about it dawns on me that I haven't had my daily dose of the comics page.

But hey, Mary Worth can wait. Our morning walk can't.

June 6, 1998

Kids, guns pose hard questions, decisions

Is it safe to send our kids to school?

That's not exactly how the father of five on the other end of the phone phrased the question, but that was the gist of it.

He'd heard that a student at a South County middle school had made some kind of threat involving upcoming graduation ceremonies.

I told him what the newspaper had learned - that a threat had been made, that security was being beefed up at the school, but that neither police nor school officials would provide any details.

And I explained that this newspaper didn't report the threat for fear that publicity would encourage copycats. He disagreed but understood our reasoning.

He went on to say that he had a high stake in all this with two children attending the school in question and three more in an elementary school. He was afraid for them, for himself and for the rest of us.

"What can we do?" he asked. "What have we come to when some hotheaded kid can get a gun and start shooting? What's to stop him? We've got to do something before we see our kids in the obituary column."

I suspect that such questions have been on the minds of parents everywhere as public schools drew to a close this week for summer vacations.

You don't have to look far or deep to see the reasons for concern. Read the headlines. Arkansas. Oregon. We see on television and in newspapers images at once horrible and fascinating. White sheets being pulled over bodies. Grief-stricken families and survivors.

The concern goes beyond the usual parental worries about a bully accosting some poor kid in a hallway for lunch money or dishing out wedgies in the locker room. Kids are getting killed by other kids armed with guns.

"It's depressing and frustrating," said Lt. Bill Stookey of the Sarasota County Sheriff's Office.

Stookey speaks of the dilemma both as a veteran law enforcement officer and father of three.

Dozens of parents called his office once the threat was known.

"We take all such threats seriously," Stookey said, adding that "99.99 percent of the time, it's a kid blowing off steam."

Some parents sought assurances that deputies were dealing with the threat. One even wanted a guarantee that nothing would happen. Another offered that anyone making such a threat "should be strung up."

"That's one thing we should have learned. Violence just begets more violence," Stookey said.

And every time it happens, we ask ourselves the same question: Why?

Round up the usual suspects: the proliferation of guns; violence on the streets, in television shows, movies and video games; broken homes; abused kids; drugs; politicians; liberals; gun nuts; and so on.

And yet we must ask ourselves: Who buys the guns?

We do.

Who patronizes the slasher-shoot-em-up movies?

We do.

Who puts the politicians in office?

We do.

I don't know the answer, but I'm inclined to agree with Lt. Stookey.

"It's gonna take all of us to address it, and we'll have to make some hard, tough decisions."

October 24, 1998

Lottery winner, give me a call

My new best friend is out there somewhere.
 I don't know if my new best friend is male or female, short or tall. In fact I don't even know what his or her name is.

But, whoever it is has a lot of money. Nearly $7 million, I figure.

Maybe you heard, and maybe you didn't, that a winning lottery ticket was sold in South Sarasota County.

To date the holder of the lucky lottery ticket has not come forward.

Here in the newsroom we've been trying to find our new best friend to no avail. We checked with the lottery office in Tallahassee and even chased rumors of parties and celebrations given for/by the lucky winner.

Of course it's possible that the lottery winner does not even live in South Sarasota County or even nearby. Who knows? Maybe the winner was a tourist who was in town playing golf or just visiting our beaches.

There's no way of knowing until the winner comes forward.

As a news story, it's less about the money than how becoming an instant millionaire changes peoples' lives. And the possibility that a new millionaire may be living among us touched off a newsroom discussion on what we would do if the state dropped $7 million in our laps.

Of course we have to pay taxes. But after that, how would you spend the money? A boat? A new car? A new house?

Should I hear from my new best friend, I would tell him/her that money is the root of all evil - or so the Bible says - and I will be happy to take some of this evil off of his/her hands.

That's just the kind of friend I am.

Said and done

I've got this new computer system in my office that's equipped with voice recognition technology.

This technology allows me to talk to a computer and it types out my words. As I've stated before, technology is a semi-wonderful thing.

This latest encounter with technology has done nothing to change my mind about that.

So I sit in my office and yap away at the computer. Occasionally, I yell at my computer screen, which it dutifully records. This makes for strange sentences, such as, "Stop that! Lowercase D—!"

Other times, it doesn't know what I want to say and ad libs. For example, when I tell the computer to write the word "million," it writes "no one" or "mill run," or some such word or words that have no meaning.

Be that as it may, for your rea`ding pleasure the following paragraphs will be dictated without the benefit of any corrections. See if you can figure out what I am trying to say.

The reason that the company got his computer is because I can no longer type. And for some strange reason they believe it or if the hair while to keep a my called.

Does that make sense to? It makes no sense to me. There are commands are the two no old to get this recognition system working properly. I guess is just going to take some time.

I now know that some things are better left on said and other things are easier down and said. To toolbar print that.

February 20, 1999

My Mother enters the computer age

Another family generation has stepped into the computer age. My mom.

We don't need much of an excuse to visit my mom.

It's not a very long drive - less than three hours by freeway, which is well within tolerable limits when accompanied by sons ages 8 and 12.

The boys are partial to Grandma's cooking - her mashed potatoes in particular. My wife enjoys her company, and even though mom and I mostly drink the same brands, her liquor seems to taste better than mine.

But there was a purpose to last weekend's visit. Mom wanted a new computer and I volunteered to help her select one, as I never pass up the chance to display my ignorance at these things when someone else is footing the bill.

Mom admits to being pretty much a novice when it comes to computer technology. A couple of years ago I gave her my old home computer, which she used to sharpen her skills at playing solitaire. And really, the computer was a clunker; no modem, and very little memory.

"I want to email my grandchildren," she confided in me.

So it was decided that the old computer would be given to a friend of mom's who would give it to another friend, who would give it to a grandson or granddaughter, and that mom would buy a new computer with all the bells and whistles.

"You'll need 64 megabytes of RAM and at least a 300 processor," I told her confidently in my best Robert Mitchum impersonation.

"Yeah right. Whatever. What's a RAM?" she asked.

"It stands for Random Access Memory," I told her, hoping she wouldn't probe further.

"What's that do?" she persisted.

"It's the kind of memory that allows you to run programs," I offered, reaching the depth of my knowledge.

"And I need 64 of them?"

"Megabytes, yes."

After church on Sunday we set out. For part of the previous night we sorted through newspaper ads for deals and sales, so we knew where to go and roughly how much she'd need to spend. We wanted a system we could carry home and set up that evening.

The first stop had nothing in her price range. At the second stop was a salesman who nearly made me feel guilty for not buying a computer that he didn't have in stock. The third stop, across the parking lot from the second, had a computer in stock within the price range, so the deal was made.

Back at the ranch, the 8-year-old unpacked the components, taking the boxes outside to construct a fort. The 12-year-old commenced hooking it up and plugging it in. It was then that we discovered the room had no phone outlet, so we couldn't engage the modem. By dinner, only the printer remained to be set up. And after a dinner of beef and mashed potatoes, we started training.

We worked for an hour or so, slogging our way through terms and concepts neither of us clearly understood. But we did get to a point where mom could write and print a letter. The email will have to wait for another day, or at least until she can get a phone line installed. I'm sure she'll be surfin' the Web soon.

And I did learn something valuable on my visit. Grandma's mashed potatoes are instant.

February 27, 1999

Dad's crooked pitch misses the plate

He bought none of it.

"Think of it as your homework," I said for the wind-up.

"No way, Dad. Washing the dishes is not part of my homework," he bunted back, emphasizing the "not."

"Extra credit then. Besides, you need to practice," I pitched.

While my 12-year-old son and I debated the merits of dishwashing, my wife had finished rinsing the dinner plates and glasses and stacked them neatly on the counter.

Only the pots and pans remained to be done.

"Dad, we do not get graded on washing dishes," the 12-year-old said firmly.

Then I threw it. High, hard and inside.

"Oh, but you do. I talk to your teacher today." I sensed his resolve dissolve.

Reluctantly, he shuffled to the sink and turned the hot water tap. My wife backed away from the sink and moved on to tackle the next in her endless stream of household tasks.

We used to call it "Home Ec," short for home economics. Because of the subject matter - cooking, sewing - it was considered a girls' class.

Today it's called "Family and Consumer Science," and it's not just for girls. The subject matter goes well beyond cooking and sewing and includes time management, budgeting money and evaluating foods for nutritional content. Most middle and high schools have a similar course.

"It's a life skills class," said Laurel Nokomis teacher Pat McCord, who noted that in one of her classes boys outnumber girls by a 4-to-1 ratio.

But, it's the cooking part of the curriculum that draws student interest.

"At this age, they love to cook. They love to be in the kitchen," McCord said.

I'm not so sure about the cooking part. But experience tells me that middle schoolers have no lack of appetite. As for them loving to be in the kitchen, well, that's where the food is.

But lets face it, kids at any age don't exactly fall over themselves volunteering to clean up. But, Ms. McCord assured me that clean-up is part of the class duties.

"Their kitchens sparkle," she said with a hint of pride in her voice.

Other practical skills are imparted to students in her class, including how to do laundry.

"We show them how to sort clothes and run a washing machine," she said.

At that point, I was ready to send flowers to Ms. McCord and nominate her for Teacher of the Year.

"What about shirts? Do you teach them how to iron shirts? And bathrooms? Can you teach them how to clean bathrooms? And windows ..."

Through my mind raced this vision of my wife and me sleeping in on Saturday mornings while the 12-year-old throws in a load of laundry and scours the bathrooms.

Then Ms. McCord burst my balloon.

No shirts, no bathrooms, no windows. No homework, either, not officially anyway.

Well, you can't have everything.

But it seems that a little hands-on housework, I mean homework, could really help kids polish their classroom skills.

April 24, 1999

Mundane moments can't be all that bad

There's been plenty of bad news to go around this week. So, to give my loyal readers - both of them - a break from the crisis in Kosovo and the killings in Littleton, Colo., here is Rich's news of the mundane from the house and neighborhood (otherwise known as column filler).

Item: Bottle Breakers Busted. A pair of 8-year-old boys were identified as the prime suspects in an incident last month in which glass bottles were broken in the street.

The broken glass was cleaned up by a conscientious neighbor. There were no injuries.

One perpetrator reached a plea bargain to perform community service - he had to pick up palm fronds; the other has not been sentenced.

The father of the boy who performed the community service was said to have been distraught over the bottle-breaking incident but proud of his son for accepting his punishment "like a man."

Item: Missing Shoe Recovered. A boy's sneaker that was missing for more than a week was discovered Tuesday when the youth's room was cleaned.

The black tennis shoe, first reported missing April 12, was found under a pile of dirty clothes. The owner of the missing shoe told authorities he feared that someone had sneaked into his room sometime between 9 p.m. April 11 and 7 a.m. April 12 and stolen the shoe.

But no witnesses reported seeing any one-legged suspects wearing a size 2 1/2 sneaker in the neighborhood that night.

The shoe was returned to service Wednesday.

Item: Wheelchair Waffles on Ramp. A motorized wheelchair became stuck on an access ramp when the wheelchair ran low on power.

The wheelchair's 46-year-old operator was rescued when his 12-year-old son manually pushed him up the ramp.

The operator had been visiting the neighbors before losing power while trying to get back to his house.

"I was luck he was nearby. I might be stuck there yet," the operator said of his rescuer, noting that he frequently turns to his son for assistance.

Item: Sheltie Sheared, Put on Diet. The owner of a 3-year-old sheltie cut the dog down to size this week, revealing girth previously covered by thick fur.

The dog reportedly was known throughout the neighborhood for his gentle disposition and abundant appetite.

The dog's owner said the sheltie would be put on a low-fat diet and pleaded with neighbors to refrain from feeding him.

Item: Yard Excavation Underway. Two boys, ages 8 and 4, started excavation operations this week in a neighbor's yard.

Using shovels and spade, the 8-year-old said they had dug past an elaborate network of roots but had not discovered any fossils, which they think will be found close to the Earth's core.

"Fossils are dinosaurs' bones, " the 8-year-old said.

And you thought all news was bad news.

June 19, 1999

Remembering dad: the good and the bad

Father's Day eve. Dads everywhere will be going to bed tonight with visions of golf clubs, power tools, neck ties and Hawaiian shirts dancing in their heads.

And, for some of us there will be memories of a father who has passed away. That's the case for me, anyway. My dad died about six years ago. And every year around this time I find myself thinking of his legacy and how his interaction with me, my two brothers and my two sisters colored by own views of fatherhood.

To wit: Sibling justice

Our house was not exactly a place of tranquility. Like most other siblings, we fought, argued and generally tried to make each other miserable. It was more of the same after lunch.

My brother two years my senior and I were the worst offenders. We would fight about nearly everything. Were hot dogs better than hamburgers? We would fight. Was ketchup better than mustard? We would fight. Was Superman cooler than Batman? We would fight.

Dad never bothered to find out which one of us was the cause of the conflict, although that question seemed of paramount importance to us. Dad's solution was to remove his belt and strap us both on our backsides, which more often than not ended the conflict. As my brother and I grew older we became accustomed to dad's discipline. All he had to do was reach for his belt buckle and the fighting stopped.

Now, I don't use a belt on either of my sons, eight and 12. But I know that it's pointless questioning the boys about the source of the argument. So, I just punish them both.

Answering the door

Dad had a way of welcoming my friends into the house. As soon as the doorbell would ring, he would holler, "Go away! We don't want any!"

The salutation often drew stares from my friends and sometimes served to scare away door-to-door salesmen.

I've adopted the same greeting with mixed results. I have managed to scare off some Jehovah's Witnesses, but the boys' friends have become immune. I now ask them if they came over to do some yard work.

Phone etiquette

Just about the time I reached the age that I wanted to call girls on the phone my dad did something to me that made me wish I had put it off for a couple more years. I was in eighth grade and finally worked up the courage to call a girl, Anne, in my class.

I dialed the number and waited patiently for her to come to the phone. Unknown to me, my dad picked up the receiver on an extension and waited for his chance.

After a few minutes of chattering away to break the ice, he struck.

"Ooof neep yorp deef," dad said into the extension.

"What was that?" Anne asked.

"Farfel ifnooya wattmacoola?" dad said.

I pleaded, "DAAAD! Get off the extension." But to no avail.

"Eeeeper fardrum hoopin gaffer!"

"That's just my dad trying to be funny," I said, but by that time Anne had hung up, figuring she was talking to a house full of kooks. I spent the better part of high school trying to convince girls that there was nothing wrong with dad other than an overactive sense of humor.

I haven't tried this on either of my two boys.

I want it to be a surprise.

July 17, 1999

4 birds in the cage worth 3 in the snake

O ur suitcases were still in the van when I heard my wife's panicky cry.

"A snake!" she screeched.

It's not uncommon to find that things around the house have changed while the family was away on vacation. Maybe the milk has spoiled, or the house plants need water.

But a 3-foot rat snake coiled around a perch in the bird cage on our back porch was more of a surprise than we bargained for.

And this was not just any snake. It was a murderer. For as we stared into its cold, unfeeling eyes, we noticed that the cage's finch population was down by three.

There's no way of knowing how long the snake had been dining on our finches. My guess is that it slithered through an opening in the screen, slipped into the cage and hid in the nest where it consumed Barb, the mother bird, and two chicks.

Every marriage has clear divisions of labor, which vary from couple to couple. For example, the husband/dad takes care of the yard and plays golf while the wife/mom takes on the laundry, cooking, cleaning and everything else.

Capturing snakes would normally be the task of the husband/dad. But because of my disabilities, the animal-control duties fell upon my bride.

So I rolled onto the porch to direct operations. Our sons, ages 8 and 13, rounded up as many neighborhood kids as possible to see Mrs. Brooks catch the snake.

Her first task was to remove the four living birds from the cage before the snake decided to look for dessert. But the birds would not cooperate. Every time she tried to capture one, it would squirm free.

This part of the operation set off a chorus of invectives from my wife punctuated by panicked screams.

It took a few minutes to round up the birds and put them in a spare cage. That done, she turned her attention to the snake.

After she donned a pair of heavy work gloves, I told my wife to pinch the snake just behind its head and pull it out of the cage. Now, dealing with snakes can be traumatic, even in cases where the snake is nonpoisonous and has a head no bigger than a finger tip.

So, I wasn't surprised when she balked at grabbing the snake, even though the gloves were probably heavy enough
to stop a .44-caliber bullet.

Every time she reached for the snake it would lunge at the gloved hand. And every time it lunged, she would scream.

"Now, just grab the snake . . ." I said. The snake lunged.

"Aaaauugghhh!" shrieked my wife.

"Try not to panic," I coached her. The snake lunged.

"Aaauugghhh!" she screamed.

This lunging-screeching pattern continued for several minutes until the snake, whether by design or sheer exhaustion, fell from the perch, landing with a thump on the bottom of the cage.

There the screeching continued as the snake, probably feeling that it was on the short end of a mismatch, tried to escape the cage. But being engorged on three birds, it was probably a few sizes larger than when it got into the cage.

She eventually caught the snake in the same net she used to catch the birds. She put the snake in a grocery sack and turned it loose near a drainage ditch.

The following morning my wife told me that she dreamed about trying to keep snakes from eating our birds. I didn't have the heart to tell her I dreamed about Col. Sanders.

October 2, 1999

The mark of a proud but annoying parent

A rare moment it was. A moment that every parent dreams of. A moment that seems to slow the march of time. A moment that energizes a lifetime. A moment that validates the sacrifices of raising children - the sleepless nights, the spit-up in the back seat of the new van, the teacher conferences.

As is usually the case with such moments, it came casually, unrehearsed - under circumstances that only served to deepen the sincerity of the gesture.

And yet there is that nagging thought, hanging in your mind like a tattered Hawaiian shirt in the back of your closet, that you should have seen it coming. Had it been a novel, it would have been recognized as foreshadowing spooned as thick as Melville in the events of the previous weekend.

Stuck at home with his dad, he was. His mother and younger brother, 8, were out of town for the weekend, so it fell upon the 13-year-old to care for his disabled father.

No easy task. But we've been through this before, and he's usually up to it.

But not even unlimited access to TV, soda pop, pizza and assorted snacks on which to graze could keep him entirely content for two days. This he expressed graciously on the afternoon of the second day.

"Dad, do you think that maybe next weekend we could, like, go to a movie or something? You know, just you and me?"

Before I could nod in agreement, he continued.

"I can't wait for Mom to get home. I mean, no offense, but you're not the easiest person to get along with. In fact, you can be real annoying. What movie do you want to see?"

Annoying? Did he say annoying?

"No offense taken," I said. He didn't hear. He was flipping through the newspaper to see what movies were playing nearby.

And so the comment slipped from the stream of his consciousness.

For me, however, his words sparked some soul searching. His point I saw clearly enough. Dressing and feeding anyone other than yourself can be a challenge. For a teenager charged with caring for his father - even if just for two days - the task can be daunting.

His words cut to the core of parenting - the ability to annoy your kids.

Then came The Moment.

While sopping spaghetti sauce with a piece of bread a couple of days later, the 8-year-old allowed that he had been invited to a friend's house to play after dinner.

The response of my wife and me was immediate. "You know the rule," I said. "No playing outside after dinner on school nights." I then continued, jokingly, or so I thought, that I had saved a bunch of chores for the 8-year-old.

With a low-grade growl and then a scream, the he let us know how he felt.

"You are so annoying, Dad," he said, his face flushed with anger. "You are the most annoying person on earth."

"He's right, Dad," said the 13-year-old, piling it on. He continued that, except for his brother, I was the most annoying person in his life.

The accolades heaped upon me were not totally lost on my wife, who flashed a huge smile and gave me a thumbs-up sign.

So it's good to know that even from a wheelchair, I can still annoy my kids.

October 30, 1999

The great dilemma of trick-or-treating

The family is getting into the Halloween spirit, so to speak.

Now I understand that even speaking of Halloween might offend some readers. And I am not condoning devil-worship, witchcraft, voodoo or any other form of magic or spell-casting to get ahead, improve study habits or repair computers.

Face it, if witchcraft worked, both Bobby Bowden and Steve Spurrier would have broken out in boils and warts long ago.

Our household's plunge into this unholy abyss is being led by the 8-year-old, whose enthusiasm for Halloween is second only to Christmas.

Several months ago he started lobbying for the family to construct some sort of haunted house for the occasion. And although my wife quickly quashed the idea, his zeal hasn't waned.

And earlier this week, when we finally got around to pulling the Halloween decorations out of the attic, it was the 8-year-old who opened the box and individually tested each prop to make sure they were all in working order.

So, the welcome mat that screams when someone steps on it and the ghost that emits an obnoxious wail when rustled by the slightest breeze are both in place and functioning according to their purpose, which is to annoy the neighbors.

We also have assorted skeletons, jack-o'-lanterns, spiders and a set of plastic chicken nuggets adorned in various costumes, sure to scare vegetarians and anyone on a low-fat diet.

But the topic that's getting the most attention is: What night do the kids go trick-or-treating?

The question became the topic of dinnertime discussion earlier this week when the 13-year-old announced that he had decided to go trick-or-treating tonight.

Silly me. I assumed that Sunday, being Halloween, would be the night for door-to-door panhandling.

"But Dad, that's a school night. We'd have to be in by 9 o'clock," he said. Then came what the 13-year-old was certain would be the clincher. "Everyone else is going Saturday night."

In the lexicon of teen-agers, "everyone" means his closest two or three friends. Suffice it to say, I was not overwhelmed by the strength of his argument.

The discussion ended when he suggested that he be allowed to trick-or-treat on both nights, a solution that was rejected.

But the question remains. Saturday would be a logical choice. It would give kids and parents a day to come down off their sugar high.

But Halloween is Sunday. Along with being a night before a school day, to many it is a day of worship. Would it be right to celebrate a pagan ritual on the Sabbath?

Heathens such as myself have no problem with that. But those who fear the fires of eternal damnation might want to stay home and leave the candy for the rest of us.

Our elected leaders could solve this problem by declaring one night or the other beggars night. After all, they have no qualms about setting aside days for just about everything else, like National Head Lice Day.

But with elections just around the corner, don't expect politicians to stick their necks out for anything this important.

Trick or treat.

December 18, 1999

How times change: joys of shopping

All the handicapped parking spaces were taken, so my wife maneuvered to the rear of the lot, where there would be plenty of room to park the van, lower the ramp and unload my wheelchair.

All week I had been looking forward to taking the boys, 8 and 13, Christmas shopping at the mall. As we approached its entrance, I thought of a time not long ago when such an outing would have filled me with dread.

I would rather have organized the garage, pull weeds or paint a closet. Cleaning fish was preferable to facing this seasonal madness.

But that was in a previous life -before I was diagnosed with Lou Gehrig's disease. Now I find shopping malls, with their open walkways, wide aisles and doorways, wonderfully accessible to those of us in wheelchairs.

I also saw it as a chance to spend time with my wife and sons.

Once inside the mall, we huddled briefly and decided to split up. My wife would go her way, and the boys would come with me. We would meet for lunch at one of the food court's five-star eating establishments.

Top on our agenda was getting gifts for my wife. With a spending limit of $10 each, the boys were squeezing their brains trying to come up with ideas.

The 8-year-old suggested a stuffed Winnie-the-Pooh or Pokemon character.

"She likes Winnie-the-Pooh," he confided.

Or how about a monster movie video or Britney Spears CD? (Coincidentally, he's partial to Godzilla and female performers.)

Sadly, neither was in his price range.

His older brother, meanwhile, was a man on a mission. He had made plans with a friend to meet for a movie inside the mall, leaving about 90 minutes to buy three gifts and, more importantly, eat lunch.

It took him only a few minutes to snare two gifts. But momentum stalled when it came to a gift for his mother. He first selected a CD single from a popular group - Counting Toes, I think was its name. The price was right, but he wondered if she would listen to a single; nor was he sure if she even liked the group.

Shopping with the boys has almost always been an enlightening experience. When they were younger, they would play hide-and-seek among racks of clothes.

We thought it was cute until a wad of gum mysteriously disappeared when one of them ducked into a row of dresses. Then there was the puppy in the pet store that looked as if an antenna was growing from behind one of its ears. "Hey, didn't you have a sucker when we came in here?" I remember asking one of the boys.

I've heard from other parents who have had similar shopping adventures. The puddle on the grocery store linoleum, the temper tantrum at the bookstore, the falling tower of cereal boxes - this is the stuff of suburban legends.

Our arms brimming with booty, we made our way through the parking lot, passing rows of Buicks, Caddies and minivans.

Security precautions prevent me from revealing exactly how the boys solved their shopping dilemma.

Sorry, honey, you'll just have to wait until Christmas.

January 15, 2000

Frustration grew as the minutes ticked away

For forty-five minutes I had been battling with my computers voice recognition software. Deadline was fast approaching and all I had the show for my labor was the date followed by this paragraph:

```
"Females and lettuce scratch that scratch that
scratch that scratch that scratch that scratch
that scratch that scratch that scratch that go
to sleep go to sleep go to sleep."
```

Figuring that it would be easier to start over, I try some voice commands to erase the lone paragraph of gibberish.

"Select paragraph," I say into the headset's microphone.

Nearly instantly, the paragraph becomes white type against a black background.

"Delete that," I say into the mike.

The text disappeared. But instead of a blank screen, the words "Believe that" appear.

"Delete that," I say again.

"Believe that," writes the computer.

I could feel the veins popping out in my neck and forehead. I'm sure my blood pressure was blowing through the roof, but I had no way of verifying that.

Exasperated, I hurl a string of obscenities into the mike.

"Kiss my airborne has you free consent of the ditch," writes the computer.

Technology is a semi wonderful thing. By nature I'm suspicious of anything that has hard drives, floppy disks, random access memory and a mouse that clicks. It seems that for each problem solved by better and faster technology new problems are created.

On the other hand, I'm probably more dependent on technology than most people. My electric wheelchair gives me mobility. An electrical lift in the family van allows me to take my wheelchair nearly anywhere. And the television remote control that many people take for granted is an essential for me. Without it I'd be unable to avail myself of the wonderful cable television lineup that includes such scintilating channels as the home shopping network, the game show channel, and the preview channel.

But I'm especially dependent on technology when it comes to writing. Lou Gehrig's disease has sapped the strength from my hands, so I can no longer operate a computer keyboard.

Technology to the rescue, sort of.

When I installed voice recognition software on my computers at home and in the office about a year ago, I thought such software would be like dictating to an efficient secretary or typist.

In reality, however, it's more like talking to an inebriated Russian who has no understanding of the English language. The software has no sense of context, grammar, or style.

And so a simple phrase such as "emails and letters," becomes "even channel sent letters" or, in the case of last week, "females and lettuce." Another example: "lacking in imagination" became "lactose" imagination.

Then there are the commands the system uses to fix booths, (I said "goofs"). For example, if it has written something that you want to remove, you say, "scratch that" into the microphone and the software deletes the phrase you have just dictated.

Or if you wish to turn off the microphone, to say, answer the phone, you'd say " Go to sleep." Sometimes, though, it writes the words instead of carrying out the command. So you can end up with the phrase repeating itself "at Nottingham," or ad nauseum.

Getting back to last week. After another forty-five minutes struggling to get one paragraph written, my wife came to the rescue. She typed while I dictated.

So when you read this column today it's more than a creative effort. It's a technological miracle.

January 22, 2000

Humor is good for heart, soul

Heard any good jokes lately?
Your health may depend on it.

I say this after having attended a daylong seminar at Selby Gardens last Saturday about treatment options for amyotrophic lateral sclerosis, or ALS, a.k.a. Lou Gehrig's disease.

For roughly four hours speakers told us of research efforts that seek the cause and cure of this disease, how the disease affects the respiratory system, and what devices are available to help ALS patients carry on.

It was pretty heavy stuff for someone such as myself who has no medical background.

As expected, all of the speakers demonstrated depth and knowledge in their respective fields.

But the show stopper came last, as if his topic, how humor plays a role in health and healing, were the desert following a heavy meal.

John L'Oreal, a professor at USF inTampa, pointed out that there's nothing humorous about disease. But, mirthful laughter can help fight sickness.

Take longer funny bone of has been shown to benefit the immune system by increasing the concentration of antibodies and increasing white blood cells in the immune system. Both of which can make the body more resistant to developing infections.

It's also been known to benefit the respiratory system the muscular system and the central nervous system.

'tis true. The beneficial effects of humor on human physiology is gaining acceptance among the medical community.

In North Carolina, for example, an organization calling itself that Carolina health and humorous initiation (Carol and a hot) to was founded in 1986. The staff of Carolina off off performs for audiences for entertainment and employee stress management programs.

But it is best known for implementing a "last mobile that is used to present humorous materials to cancer patients at the Duke University medical center.

The last mobile is a roving cart equipped with books, tapes, and gains, videos and props such as rubber chicken zeal using water guns.

Other humor intervention programs have popped up in hospitals in Phoenix San Diego, Philadelphia, Dallas and Brooklyn.

At Sarasota Memorial hospital Carlos the Clown visits patients and appears at public functions.

So, in keeping with the theme of today's column, and because I still need to fill a few more inches, how close with a joke lifted from an Internet site about psychological humor.

Two guys are sweeping in a warehouse and suddenly one guy starts climbing up the side of the wall and when he gets to the top starts shouting "I'm a light bulb." The manager comes in and see this and tells him to get down and get back to work. After 20 minutes the same guy does the same act. The manager this time warns him that if he does it again he will be fired and to stop it. Twenty minutes later he is up there again; the manager says, "That's it you're fired, get out of here." The man climbs down from the ceiling and starts to walk out and the other man starts out after him. The manger asks the second man where he thinks he is going and the man says, "I'm not working in the dark."

March 18, 2000

It's a home invasion

With his elbows propped up on sand bags, the major squinted through field glasses.

The defenses, he saw, were manned and in place. At the same time, a lieutenant snapped a salute to a grimy brow and reported the same. "All units report ready, sir."

"Very well," the major nodded. He fumbled with the cap to his canteen, and silently wished for a shot of the 12 year old Scotch he kept in his liquor cabinet for special occasions.

"That'll have to do," he said gulping down a slug of stale water.

To the West, the sun was dipping behind some cumulous clouds that had gathered over the horizon. From somewhere behind him in the compound he heard the lilting song of the tufted titmouse. He glanced at his watch. Seventeen hundred hours.

Soon, he thought, very soon.

His troops would be in for the fight of their lives. Young and green, the major privately wondered if there
were up to the task.

"Sir, radar reports three contacts," came a voice from inside a nearby bunker.

If the major was nervous, he didn't show it. His steel blue eyes narrowed; his teeth clenched. "Radio all units to stand by and hold their positions," he said evenly.

"Alpha sector reports... sorry sir I can't make it out it sounds like..." the radio operator's voice trailed off.

"Minivan at eleven o'clock," barked the lieutenant. "We've got uncles and cousins at the perimeter." The major lifted his field glasses in time to see a white Caravan slowing to a halt.

"Beta reports an SUV closing on their position from the Northwest," the radio operator shouted.

"Good gravy!" shouted the major. "It's a Suburban! They've got toddlers! Tell Beta Company to fall back and rendezvous..."

"A nephew has broken through the perimeter and is coming up the driveway, " shouted the lieutenant.

The major had been ready for that. "Put the beer cooler in the driveway. That will slow his advance." He knew that twist off caps would be too easy, so he opted for the old-style bottles, hoping that the search for an opener would buy more time.

The major's bunker provided a clear view of the carnage that was about to take place in the driveway. Behind the nephew, an aunt and grandmother had broken through the defenses and were now encircling alpha company.

"Fall back! Fall back!" the major yelled. But it was too late. The aunt and grandmother had captured the nine-year-old.

"They're kissing him! I can't watch," said the lieutenant. The major knew this was the beginning of the end.

"We've got two brothers-in-law and a brother assaulting her the front gate. There are also reports of cousins and sisters in that group," said the radio operator.

That would be the main assault force, the major thought to himself and wondered how long the would be before they reached his position.

If they succeeded in crashing through the front, it would be a straight shot to the...

"The liquor and drinks are all set up," said my wife.

A pair of electronic tones sounded from the speakers inside the compound. The major closed his eyes as if trying to forestall the inevitable.

"Would someone please answer the door?" my wife asked the 13 year old. "It's not polite leaving relatives standing on the porch."

The lieutenant jumped from the bunker. "Honey, your family's here. How long are you going to sit there and stare out the window?"

But the major didn't move. He would not surrender. They would never take him alive.

April 22, 2000

Wheelchairs crimp restaurant dining

With an arched eyebrow, he uttered a string of obscenities loud enough to be heard above the din of the bar. His face had gone from a healthy tan to a shade of red with violent highlights.

From my wheelchair I witnessed this transformation, which started right after the hostess told us we would have to wait 45 minutes to an hour for a table.

We had made reservations, knowing that eating at a popular restaurant on Friday night would draw both tourists and locals. The tables were ready when our party began to arrive.

Then I showed up in my wheelchair.

A young man with blond hair and earring told us that no one had told them to expect someone in the wheelchair. As a result, they seated us in a part of the restaurant inaccessible to wheelchairs.

So, we waited and sipped drinks at the bar while my friend fumed. I wasn't too upset because he was buying the drinks. His mistake had been to go out to eat with someone who needs a wheelchair to get around.

In the two or so years I've needed a wheelchair, I've come to look at such experiences as inconvenient obstacles. I keep track of those places that are easily accessible and those that are not, patronizing the former and avoiding the latter.

Sometimes, though, there is no choice, just as there are some obstacles that are easier to overcome than others. Most restaurants are equipped with ramps and doors wide enough for wheelchairs. Once inside, though, people in wheelchairs find themselves asking diners to move their chairs because there's not enough room to maneuver between tables.

That's manageable. But imagine having to meet your boss or client for lunch only to find out that the restaurant is on the second floor of a building that has no elevators. What do you do? Order carry out?

Steps, doors that only open one-way, aisles and doorways too narrow for a wheelchair are just some of the physical barriers that must be overcome.

And there are plenty of such places around, including a bar in Sarasota where my college alumnus gather to watch football games. There are no ramps there, only steps. More than once I've been lifted, wheelchair and all, to get inside. And, there's the religious bookstore named for the patron saint of hopeless causes. But if you're in a wheelchair, you can't go inside because there's no ramp.

An acquaintance who's been in a wheelchair for most of his adult life told me of waiting in a men's restroom for better than 20 minutes until someone opened the door for him from the outside. One woman whose husband has had a stroke complained to me of a restroom in a doctors office that has no grab-bars. Being elderly, she isn't strong enough to hold him up. And without the grab bars he can't use the bathroom alone.

Traveling with a wheelchair can be an adventure. In half dozen or so hotels I've stayed at since being wheelchair-bound, only one had a shower that could accommodate a wheelchair. All the others had bathtubs. Want to know what it's like for someone in a wheelchair to get into and out of a bathtub? Tie your ankles together and try it!

Thankfully, there are many buildings – museums, most public venues, shopping malls, even stadiums – that make getting around in wheelchairs easy. Ramps are clearly marked, aisles are wide, shop doors are open, restrooms are not blocked by one-way doors, and there are grab bars in the stalls.

Such accommodations can really make the difference for people with physical handicaps.

They shouldn't have to worry about whether they will get stuck in the restroom. And, there are more important things to think about – like getting someone else to pay for my drinks.

July 22, 2000

Family games illuminates competition

As we approached, we saw the playing surface illuminated by fluorescent lights.

"Time to put on the game face, "I said to the nine-year-old as we came to the edge of the counter top.

I raised the seat of my wheelchair and the nine-year-old, my assistant, pulled up a chair. On the counter was the game board, built on a lazy Susan so that it could pivot.

The other players, the 14 year old and my wife, took positions around the game board. The 14 year old was confident of victory. A cocky smirk crossed his lips as he sized up the opposition. Certain he was that his middle-aged father and mother couldn't match his skill.

He had reason to be confident. None of his friends had been able to defeat him.

But the opposition this night were not teenagers.

Like him, we were readers. We preferred books, magazines and newspapers to most anything that appeared on the screen. Just a week before, the 14 year old plowed through the 700 pages of the latest Harry Potter book in less than three days.

And let's face it, few games test your vocabulary like Scrabble.

For all of our bravado, at least on the part of the 14 year old and myself, we were really not very good at this game. Most of our words are of the three-letter variety. Words of two or more syllables are about as common as goals in a pro soccer game.

But this was not about winning or losing, although any game sparks a certain competitive spirit. This was "Family Game Night."

At the suggestion of a friend we decided to try this as a way to relate to each other without the baggage of being a father/decision maker/disciplinarian or a mother/nurturer/disciplinarian.(Our actual titles are "Czar" for me and "The Boss" for my wife.)

the original idea was for the family to gather around a game one evening a week. But that schedules never really developed. Finding a time when the boss was not exhausted and the czar was not too tired was difficult.

Furthermore, the nine-year-old, who acts is my assistant because my hands don't work, can be, well, stubborn and unwilling, traits inherited from the boss's side of the family. In addition, he is not quite at the age where he enjoys playing board games, although he once had the idea to challenge Bill Gates to a game of Candyland for all of Gates' money.

But after he was threatened with solitary confinement, he became a reluctant assistant.

The game started with the 14 year old putting down the letters F-I-G. From my prospective, it was not a word.

"Gif? What is a gif?" I said.

"Dad," said the 14 year old in exasperated tone, "you're looking at the board upside-down."

He didn't recognize a ploy designed to crack his concentration.

On my turn, I added the letters U-R-E to FIG and jumped to the early lead.

After an hour of play, space and letters were at a premium. So I fell back on a trusted tactic –make up words.

"Bolu is not a word, Dad," the 14 year old challenged.

"Yes it is," I said. "It's what the monkey guy said to James Franciscus in the movie, 'Valley of the Gwange.' "

My wife, who vowed more than 20 years ago to support me for better or worse and all that, sided with the 14 year old.

Not that I needed the help. The czar defeated all, causing much consternation to 14 year old.

"So what will we play next week?" I prodded the 14 year old.

"I don't know," said he. "I need to find a game I can beat you at."

That will be a cold day in lleh.

August 5, 2000

Exploring the different meanings of growth

Growth is a word with many conflicting connotations. To some, growth means business. It means new customers moving into an area. This can be good or bad, depending on your point of view.

For teenagers, a growth can be that mutated blob on your neck or forehead striving to become a new life form, or maybe it's just a zit.

For parents, however, growth is what happens to your kids when you're not paying attention. Child-rearing experts point out that growth for humans is uneven. They seem to grow by leaps and bounds, as opposed to a steady rate.

And some growth doesn't stop, even after your spirit has passed on to greater rewards, or eternal damnation, depending on how much fun you had in your lifetime. Did you know that your hair continues to grow after you are dead? This explains why corpses dug up in B-movies always seem to be having bad hair days.

This growth has many ramifications. For example, aunts, uncles, and grandmothers who have not seen your kids for a few months will almost certainly remark on how they have grown. This will be followed by a sloppy kiss from the aunt who has a hairy mole the size of a peach pit on her upper lip.

Shopping for back to school clothes and shoes is where kids' growth becomes most apparent.

For it is during these family excursions that parents learn the T-shirts you bought in the spring no longer cover your kid's navel, although said offspring will surely insist that it fits just fine, which would be true if he were a belly dancer.

And shoes? You know your teenager has grown when you find yourself shopping for his school shoes at a boat marina. "Do you have Boston Whalers in size 12 1/2 triple E?"

Of course, not all growth is physical. Believe it or not, their brains expand as well and they become more intellectually astute and mature.

Now, this phenomenon may not become noticeable until the kid reaches roughly 13 or 14. I know parents past and present marvel at how kids went from being inquisitive 12-year-olds who wonder why this sky is blue to teenagers who know virtually everything.

And in just one year! What is even more astounding is that this has been accomplished without the budding reference section even cracking a serious book or watching the Discovery Channel. Nooooo! This intellectual earthquake occurred while they were watching MTV and playing video games.

I am not flying solo in this salient observation. Having conversed at length with fellow experts in teenager-hood (okay, so I talked with some other parents of teenagers), I have concluded that my conclusions are confirmed.

"I don't know how I got with this far without having a teenager to consult," said Gary, who has two teens living at his home.

"What did I ever do before we had a teenager and the house?" remarked Jeff, father of two.

The teens themselves take all this in stride. They are unfazed by the sudden change in their intellectual capacity and accept it with nonchalant confidence.

And yet, the sudden onset of smarts does not seem to have affected their vocabulary, because only one word is used to answer any query by a parent. That word is, "Duh."

So, how did they become so smart in such a short period of time? By excluding other more conventional forms of learning, such as hard work, study, reading and attending lectures, we come up with one theory that fits the facts as we know them: osmosis.

Yes, the chemical action that allows a smell to dissipate throughout a room is the same action that allows teenagers to become smart by not doing anything. They just need to watch MTV and play video games while knowledge seeps into their cranium.

To bad it's not that easy for the rest of us.

Duh!

September 25, 2000

Slipping in and out of the digital age

"Don't eat with your fingers!," I said to the nine-year-old. He complied with my half hearted admonition, lowering his hand and clutching his fork.

Kids certainly need to practice good manners. My mother lived with the fear that I would be wearing underwear admitted into a hospital emergency room unless I was wearing clean underwear. My fear is that my sons will dig their fingers into the mashed potatoes or double dip into the pate while dining out with a girl or, worse, her parents.

Yet, it's only natural – using hands, I mean.

And I'm pretty sure that the nine-year-old, his reasoning skills uncluttered by notions of etiquette and manners, understands that. In his world, where the links between cause and effect are clear and immediate, forks, knives and spoons are extraneous redundancies of perfect tools: our hands.

We know that the opposing thumb allows us to manufacture tools and accomplish a host of other tasks that separate us from other species.

Metaphors of gripping and grasping hands fill our language. Have you lost your grip? Do you have a good grasp of the facts? Lend a hand to a friend. Performers live to receive a hand from the audience. Some say they can measure character by the strength of a handshake: a firm grip is good, a limp handshake is not. Would that it should be so easy.

Its nearly impossible to overstate the hand grip's significance to humanity. Individually, however, it's easy to take it for granted.

This I share with the nine-year-old. We are both eager to use our hands. He because every instinct tells him that working hands are a gift. Me because my hands no longer work.

Even though amyotrophic lateral sclerosis –ALS, also known as Lou Gehrig's disease – took this gift from my grasp, the family has helped me adjust.

This adjustment is most evident at meal time. Dad-feeding duties fall most heavily upon my wife. However, the nine-year-old and his 14 year old brother pitch in.

This has made for some interesting moments.

One such moment comes each Saturday when the 14 year old and I are left home by ourselves, forced to watch college football games, drink soda, consume chili dogs, salsa and chips.

Being a devoted fan, the 14 year old does not like to avert his eyes from the action on television. Unfortunately, this detracts from his ability to land food safely in my mouth. So, chili dogs, accompanied by cheese, chopped onions and mustard, occasionally crash into my nose or upper lip.

The nine-year-old has his own method. Perpetually in a hurry to finish eating so he can play outside, he has little patience for people such as myself who need to chew their food. He handles feeding duties as one would toss tree branches into a wood chipper.

For my wife, the difficulty is navigating the fork between the plate and my mouth. Thus, my shirt and trousers often bear witness to what I had, or didn't have, for lunch or dinner.

Then there are those times when my wife uses her hands to supplement the meal time discussion with animated gestures.

She waves the fork around while I lunge and snap at it when it passes close to my face.

My wife can testify that there are hazards. Once, she held out some french fries. I chomped. She yelped, "My finger!"

"I thought it was a French fry," I said.

The foods I miss most? Finger foods, of course.

And yes, you could say I've lost my grip.

December 30, 2000

Remembering the reasons for the holidays

There is a scene in the movie "Mutiny" in which a soldier is kneeling at his bunk, his eyes closed and his hands folded in prayer.

"What are you praying for?" another soldier asks.

"I'm not praying for anything," came the reply. "I'm just giving thanks."

I hope the movie's producers forgive me for not getting the lines exactly right, but the video had to be returned to avoid paying late fees. But, that is roughly the gist of it.

The scene lasted for perhaps 30 seconds, and yet I found it clinging to my memory last week as I scoured malls and department stores with my sons, 14 and 10, seeking an appropriate gift for my wife.

To me, the movie scene presented a contrast. Here was a man who faced death in his daily duties. Yet, the found enough in his life to kneel and give thanks for what he had.

The holidays, too, present such contrasts.

Many of us celebrate the season with
music, parties and gift giving. Kids are out of school, which the gives them the chance to break in, or simply break, new toys.

For Christians, the reason for the celebration is the birth of the Christ child, yet the season itself is steeped in our pagan heritage which celebrated the winter solstice.

Still, there are many who have little reason to make merry.

While parents such as myself sometimes worry whether our children liked the gifts we gave them, there are parents who can ill afford to give their kids any new toys or clothes.

There are the aged living in nursing homes forgotten by their families and friends. There are the chronically ill who face the thought that this day might be their last. There are the mentally ill whose tortured emotions and thoughts bankrupt reality. There are working families who must decide between paying a medical bill or repairing the car that takes them to work.

The pages of this newspaper are filled with such contrasts.

We report about new homes and developments, as well as those who sleep under overpasses or in cardboard boxes.

We tell of the triumphs of peace, and war in the Holy Land.

We report breakthroughs in medicine, and tell of those who cannot afford health insurance. Our sports pages are devoted to athletes whose feats seem almost super human. And in news pages we tell of those who can no longer walk, or whose bodies are sustained by feeding tubes and respirators.

In our food pages, we offer readers recipes to create sumptuous feasts. And yet, we see news reports of children starving in faraway lands whose names seem to fall together in some strange recurring nightmare.

Our critics reveal for us writers, actors and musicians whose artistic insight seems to provide a glimpse of the wisdom or truth

And there are those for whom the truth is something to be manipulated for personal gain.

These were the thoughts I had as I maneuvered my wheelchair through crowds of shoppers while trying to find an appropriate gift for my wife. I know there are others who have the same problem I have shopping for the woman of the house. She has few interests outside her family and her job. She has no hobbies, doesn't play golf or like power tools. I point this out to demonstrate how much easier it is to buy gifts for men. A new putter, or a circular saw works just fine for them.

So, the boys and I bought her a toaster oven.

A toaster oven isn't the most sentimental gift for someone who means so much to us. But, I figured that at least she would find this gift useful.

Our booty collected, we headed through the parking lot to the van. The boys were elated that the task was completed while I felt much like the soldier praying in the barracks – grateful for all that my wife and I have.

So take stock of your heart and soul as the new year approaches.

And if all you need is a toaster oven, then you have much to be thankful for.

May 5, 2001

Reaching a state of denial

My wife and I are news junkies. We read newspapers, watch network news shows each day and tune in to CNN and SNN to keep up with events nationally and locally.

Like other journalists, I consider keeping up with news to be part of my job. My wife considers being informed an act of good citizenship. (We also read Mary Worth, but that's another story.)

Our news Jones is a stark contrast to our friend, who avoids news as if it were some communicable disease. Her outlook makes for some interesting encounters when she travels from her home in the midwest to visit us in Florida.

Even so, I was stunned at her behavior during one visit when my wife and I turned to network TV news broadcast.

As soon as the anchor began delivering the top story, our friend cupped her hands to cover her ears and started yelling, "La la la la," to drown out the anchor.

Her childish behavior made me furious, and I told her as much.

After all, I thought, here was a grown, college educated professional woman acting like a six-year-old. Her defense was that the news was all " bad news." It was as though she believed creating a state of denial would somehow made the controversies and tragedies of the world disappear.

Those of us in the news business hear this complaint from readers and viewers pretty frequently. We address it by balancing our coverage of crime, taxes, growth and politics with "brights" – uplifting stories focusing on the good things people do.

I caught myself thinking about my friend and her la la defense this week while reading an article comparing the effects of different respiratory therapies on patients with Lou Gehrig's disease, a degenerative terminal illness. As many of you know, I have Lou Gehrig's disease, a.k.a. amytrophic lateral sclerosis (ALS), so my interest in this article was more than casual.

In the article, Dr. Hiroshi Mitsumoto, director of the Eleanor and Lou Gehrig MDA/ALS Center at Columbia Presbyterian Medical Center in New York, said that many people with ALS avoid discussing end-of-life issues with their doctors and families.

The article made it clear to me that I, too, live in a State of Denial.

With good reason. I doubt if there is anyone facing a serious and/or terminal illness or injury who doesn't need some sort of denial mechanism to forge through daily living.

If Dr. Mitsumoto is to be believed, we cram our consciousness with other thoughts, maybe even meditations or prayers. This is the equivalent of covering our ears and chanting "La la la!" at the top of our lungs to drown out the sound of our lives slipping away.

This way we can maintain at least a facade of sanity, allowing us to meet with teachers, attend seminars, recitals, soccer games, watch football on television, and smile politely at lame jokes.

Like my friend who refuses to read newspapers or watch Peter Jennings, sometimes the bad news intrudes on our sheltered version of reality.

Carbon dioxide and other fossil fuel byproducts are heating the earth's atmosphere, but there's no reason to cut carbon dioxide emissions.

La la la!

Florida Legislature passes a huge tax cut, but our public schools are among the nation's worst.

La la la!

My neck muscles are getting weaker, making it more difficult to hold my head up.

La la la!

It's possible that scientists and medical researchers will find cures and treatments for cancer, heart disease, Alzheimer's, ALS and other afflictions. When that happens, I'll be glad to leave The State of Denial forever. I'm sure others will, too.

May 12, 2001

Mother's day: Who loves ya, baby?

Dear Mom,
 I started out trying to write a column about Mother's Day and the meaning of motherhood.

I thought better of it, however. Writing about peoples relationships with their mothers is sort of like chasing chickens or hearding cats – it's a complex and deeply personal subject.

So, I decided to focus on the only mother I have – you.

Naturally, this journey took me to my own childhood.

One of my most enduring memories is of all the squabbles and bickering among we five kids. Strangely, I have almost no recollections of you yelling at us or losing your temper.

As I am now the father of two active boys, 10 and 15, I see how kids test one's patience. How did you do it?

Growing up as the fourth of five children did have its advantages, however.

One such advantage was having two older brothers, Doug and Ray, plow the ground ahead of me. Because all of us attended the same elementary school and high school, the lay teachers, nuns and priests knew what to expect.

Furthermore, there was no pressure on me to over achieve, thanks largely to my brothers' academic records.

And I didn't. I can now confess that I didn't strive for better grades in order to maintain the sense of camaraderie and duty I felt to my siblings. I didn't want them to feel bad. Achieving the honor roll or becoming a Fulbright scholar would have crushed their fragile egos.

Do you think your two elder sons would have been as successful – one the vice president of an international building materials company, the other an investment banker – had I not sacrificed myself at the altar of academic mediocrity?

This may come as a surprise to you, but our household was not exactly a picture of serenity.

I remember Dad once likened our family to the Cleavers of "Leave It to Beaver." My memory is a little fuzzy, but I think he said something to the effect that we would be just like the Cleavers, "if Wally and the Beaver were from Hades." (Actually, I think he used stronger language. Such salty talk was a rarity for Father, wasn't it?)

Of course, there were dozens of trips to the emergency room to stitch gashes and set broken bones.

How you managed to maintain such an even keel through all this still amazes me.

Because Doug was only two years my senior, he and I developed a fierce sibling rivalry that occasionally erupted into fisticuffs. We locked horns over whether Popeye was tougher than Bluto, whether ketchup tasted better than mayonnaise, and whether his friends were nicer than my friends

Yet it seems you never raised your voice.

I recall fondly such moments as the time I locked myself in the bathroom to keep Doug from breaking open my head wound after the stitches had been removed . My psychotherapist told me that while such bittersweet memories may never go away, the proper medication can help me cope.

Now we are both grown with families of our own, separated by only 1,100 miles.

Looking back, I marvel at how you sustained your composure through all of these familial tribulations.

You set a pretty high standard for parenting and hope to learn your secret some day. You really are terrific. Happy Mother's Day!

Love,
Richard

PS I hope that the gift we sent didn't break during shipping. I hate to think of all that good whiskey going to waste!

August 18, 2001

Parenthood and the power to annoy

Parenting has a pretty steep learning curve.

"It gets better," I remember being told by my brother-in-law, a physician, after the birth of our first son more than 15 years ago.

Like many first-time parents, we were overwhelmed by a cute, cuddly bundle of smiles and coos. But his sleeping habits, or lack thereof, drained my wife's reservoir of patience.

Coming home one day from a 6 a.m. to 3 p.m. shift at a Southern California daily, I was once greeted by my wife still dressed in her bath robe.

"Here's your son," she announced through clenched teeth while holding the baby at arm's-length. She then marched into the bedroom for some needed rest.

My brother-in-law's prediction was partly true. The challenges of having an infant in the house were replaced by others – toilet training, sleeping through the night, homework, etc.

As they grow, childrens' attitudes toward their parents evolve as well. Until they are roughly 8 years old, kids think the world of their parents and seek parental affirmation in nearly everything they do.

By the time they become teenagers, this evolutionary cycle turns 180 degrees. Experts insist that teenagers still want the approval of their parents. Outwardly, however, parents are treated like lepers. Responses to parental queries take the form of sneers and conversations are reduced to a series of grunts: one for yes, two for no.

At this stage, developing new methods to annoy and embarrass your children is vital to their psychological well-being.

Some misguided parents may be squeamish about treating their children this way, believing its better to give their sons or daughters unqualified love and support as they test their wings of independence.

I suggest those parents conduct a memory exercise to bolster their fortitude for this task.

Think of those sleepless nights you suffered through when they were infants. Think of the time he decided to test the absorption power of his "big kid" underpants in the canned soup section of the supermarket. Remember that phone call from the teacher who revealed that your academically above-average offspring hasn't done any homework for a month? "I dunno," was the reason.

Of course, parents are not obligated to find activities with the sole purpose of annoying your kids. But, if there is something you enjoy and it annoys your teenager, consider it a happy coincidence.

Music often provides such an activity. It's been my experience that today's teenagers are about as fond of baby boomers taste in music as were the parents of baby boomers.

I learned this last week when my wife and I took a rare shopping excursion together, without the lights of our lives – our 15 year old son and his ten-year old brother.

We loped carefree among the department store's wide aisles and thumbed with unabashed pleasure through music CDs, settling on a collection of Motown hits (for just $6).

Arriving home, we cranked up the stereo to Junior Walker, Gladys Knight, Smokey Robinson, the Four Tops, the Temptations and Little Stevie Wonder.

The 15-year-old's protest was inaudible as Gladys Knight's version of "Heard It through the Grapevine" rattled the bookcase.

"Tumph ripth glowmff," he declared and stalked out of the room to catch the screaming banshees on MTV's "Total Request Live."

If Motown elicits this kind of response, imagine what The Beach Boys can accomplish.

November 17, 2001

Following the path of Lou Gehrig

On July 4, 1939 baseball great Lou Gehrig stood before a crowd at Yankee Stadium and said he was "the luckiest man alive."

In many ways, the speech by the Yankee first baseman, a lifetime .340 hitter known as "The Iron Horse," has become a testament to courage in the face of adversity. Instead of complaining about the disease he had been diagnosed with, he used his speech to recount what a terrific life he had and that he was thankful for it.

Two years later, Gehrig died of the disease that now bears his name.

There are two reasons for me to now recall Gehrig's famous speech. First, I don't have the great Gehrig's batting average, but I have his disease.

Secondly, with Thanksgiving just a few days away, it's a good time to take stock of the many things we have for which to be thankful.

It has been more than six years since I was diagnosed with amyotrophic lateral sclerosis (ALS), an affliction that gradually destroys the neurons that connect the brain with muscle tissue. Over the course of the disease, muscles become useless and atrophied. The disease has no known cause and no cure; 80 percent of its victims die within five years of diagnosis.

Which brings me to my first point: I am glad to be here.

Having a debilitating disease has helped me understand that good health and life are gifts to be cherished.

Now, this does not mean that I go through each day in a perpetual haze of spiritual bliss. With two sons, ages 15 and 11, two dogs, a yard filled with weeds and garage in constant need of cleaning, I have ample opportunities for frustration.

Yet, having to occasionally ask the teenager to lift me into my wheelchair, and having to ask No. 2 son to help feed me means that I must temper my demands and be more forgiving of shortcomings or errors.

My kids will probably tell you that I could do better in this area, and they are right. I am equally certain that they will use this paragraph against me the next time I make them pull weeds or clean the garage.

To which I will reply, "Don't believe everything you read."

Which brings me to my second point: I am thankful for having such a terrific family, friends and co-workers. Without them, I would not be able to perform even the simplest tasks.

Certainly, this illness has extracted a toll on myself and those around me. Where I once played golf, softball and other sports, now I get around using an electric wheelchair. I can no longer feed, dress or bathe myself.

At home, I rely on my wife and sons. At work, I depend on my co-worker Phyllis Breeden to feed me and occasionally get my coffee.

This dependence on others is perhaps the most frustrating element of this disease. It is frustrating because we are all trained to be independent. From the time we are infants, we are prepared to become self-sufficient.

But our independence and self-sufficiency is an illusion.

Through this disease I have come to understand that we're all dependent on another in many different ways. Our lives are interconnected, just as those leaves of the oak tree are connected to its roots.

For me, this dependence is at the surface and obvious at all times.

Though you can walk, talk, write a letter, hold a baby, shake hands, swallow food or drink bourbon without a straw, you are still dependent on others.

Which brings me to my final point: in the act of giving thanks, we will gather with family and friends to partake in a traditional feast.

Take the time this week to celebrate our dependence and in doing so, count your blessings. I have no doubt you'll find that they are many.

October 19, 2002

A family that works together is better able to work things out together

The 16-year-old stormed into his room, slamming the door behind him.

At the time, I was tempted to reprise a Groucho Marx line: Don't leave in a huff. Wait and leave in a minute-and-a-huff.

But, seeing my wife glowering at me from the kitchen, where she stood over a sink piled high with dirty dishes, I thought better of it. This was not a time for humor.

What happened next, I could have predicted based on experience. She began putting away the stack of pots and pans that had been gathering in the drainer by the sink. This she accomplished with as much crashing and slamming as possible, just in case I missed the not-so-subtle hints that she was upset with me.

I was angry too. From my perspective, though, my response, and that of my oldest son, was expected.

Having grown up in a family with two older brothers and two sisters, one younger and one older, I am familiar with familial clashes. They are part of a normal family's developmental landscape. This applies to clashes among siblings as well as parent-offspring relationships.

Above the phone in the house of my childhood, there was a postcard-size sign that read: "I consider the day a total loss unless I catch hell from someone." My older sister scratched out the word "someone" and wrote in "daddy."

As my role model for fatherhood, I guess you could say the handwriting was on the wall.

My wife, on the other hand, grew up in a household with just her older sister and mother. They had conflagrations, too, although they were less frequent and didn't usually take the form of hand-to-hand combat, as was the norm at my childhood household.

While few of our experiences prepared us for parenting in an age of cable television, Internet chat rooms and mindless video games, there are some lessons from a few generations ago that are still relevant today.

On the family farm, the foundation of the rural-agricultural economy around the turn of the last century, the success of the household required that all members of the family – sons, daughters, fathers, mothers –helped shoulder the work.

My father handed down stories of how he and his 10 siblings "slopped the chickens and milked the hogs" around the house and the small farm he grew up on.

I'm sure others have heard similar stories from their parents, grandparents or great-grandparents, an indication that such experiences were pervasive.

I suspect that these tasks helped give children an identity and sense of belonging. By performing essential jobs, kids could see their importance to the family well-being. This probably increased the esteem in which parents held their children. Following this thread, it's not a great leap to suggest that this relationship helped cool tempers during family squabbles.

Why? Well, it was probably difficult for farmer dad to hold a grudge against his teenage son if he needed that same son to plow the south forty.

Which brings me to the present, the 16-year-old, myself, and our respective temper tantrums. Looking back, I can't recall what the disagreement was about. I do know that after half an hour or so, I called on the 16-year-old to lift me from my reclining chair into my wheelchair, one of several tasks he and his 11-year-old brother perform for their father a couple of dozen times a week.

It's not plowing the south forty, but it is essential to my family. And, it is difficult to hold a grudge against someone who bears such a weight.

And although parents may find it easier to do the dishes or other household tasks themselves, they owe it to their kids to delegate as much as possible.

Your children's happiness depends on it.

January 11, 2003

Forray into parochial school proves scary

At the beginning of this school year, our younger son was attending a local parochial school. He did not want to be there, but being the tough soul that he is, he was willing to leave his friends in public schools, believing that his parents decision was best.

Chief among his concerns was that we had enrolled him in a daily religion class. Having been immersed in the dogma of the Baltimore catechism by Franciscans as a youngster myself, I was fairly confident that academic exposure to religion would stretch his mind.

I was right, but not in the way I had originally wanted.

The 12-year-old displayed qualities of linear thinking that would have made any philosophy professor proud.

This skepticism revealed itself to my wife and I shortly after the first week of classes.

"How is religion class?" I queried as we rode home from the bus stop one afternoon.

"Weird," said he.

The details were sketchy, but the gist of his story was that during a religion class another teacher had stepped in and told the students that she had seen a "vision" of Mary, the mother of Jesus, floating near a tree.

From his demeanor, I could tell he was troubled by her account.

"It was scary," he said. "It was like a ghost."

"Did you believe her?" I prodded.

He rolled his eyes. "There's no such thing as ghosts," he declared.

Then, he turned the tables with his own interrogation. How can a teacher believe in such things?

Suddenly, I felt like the fat kid in a playground game of dodgeball.

I started telling him that in matters of faith and religion, sometimes people believe in things they can't see, or even prove they exist. My answer did not satisfy him. This I knew because of that faraway look in his eyes as he gazed out the window.

Fortunately, the van pulled into our driveway before he finished reloading. Praise be to St. Thomas Aquinas, I muttered to myself.

The 12-year-old is not unfamiliar with religious concepts. He's even been known to pray, seeking High Power indulgences for such things as a go cart for himself and a cure for me.

Still, his questions infused me with a dose of guilt, attributable to my Roman Catholic upbringing. I probably would have found it easier to answer biological questions about the birds and the bees.

I'm probably not alone in preferring to field questions of biology to theology.

Science, with its step-by-step process, testing and retesting, is a method that offers proof to questions.

In theology the proof is the faith. It does not stand to scientific testing because the essence of faith is spiritual, and is not bound by the laws of physics or biology. One either accepts the faith or doesn't. There is no method for proof.

Science and religion coexist in our world, occupying different planes of thought in an uneasy truce. Societies that filter everything through a religious lens run the risk of stagnating politically, economically and morally. One needs to look no further than the Muslim-based theocracies in the Middle East for proof of this.

Where permitted to thrive, both science and religion invite us to examine deeper questions of who we are and where we came from.

We may never answer these questions. But, clues can be found in the double-helix of the human gene, and perhaps in prayers of a 12-year-old boy.

March 1, 2003

Lion and saint: saying goodbye to Two-Drink Betty

Wisps of snow blew across the parking lot of St. Andrews church as we pulled in behind the hearse.

My face and hands stung from the cold as my 17-year-old son lowered my wheelchair. In silence I followed the tracks in the snow made by the gurney bearing mom's casket, noting that the cold and sobering weather seemed appropriate for the occasion.

Funerals, it is said, are a chance for the living to say goodbye. They provide a bridge to reflect upon the passage of a life; as if by contemplating the flow of eternity, we can understand the finality of death.

Death came suddenly to Mary Elizabeth Brooks Feb. 11, shocking those of us who had come to depend on her always *being there*. She was 86.

Eulogies have a way of turning their subjects into either lions or saints. Mom was a bit of both, and a lot of neither. She was unflappable, witty, astute, intelligent and spiritual, but not pious. Her gentle blue eyes belied the heart of a warrior. She liked Elvis Presley, Canadian whiskey, golf and bridge.

We grew up, two brothers, two sisters and myself, in an unremarkable neighborhood in Columbus, Ohio during an unremarkable era.

A traveling salesman, dad was on the road for much of the year. In his absence, mom acted as the family CEO, judge, jury and resident monarch.

And she could dance.

At an eighth-grade graduation party for my oldest brother Raymond, mom and Ray entered a dance contest. Dancing the jitterbug to Elvis' "All Shook Up," they took first place.

When a priest threatened to expel Ray for allegedly cheating on an essay exam, she noted that there was no evidence except that the accused scored higher than expected on the test. Mom confronted the priest and Ray was retested with the priest watching. The score was the same; the accused exonerated; and the priest, who mom later described as a "pompous jerk," embarrassed.

We siblings were encouraged, but not pressured, to participate in sports and other activities. The caveat was that we had to find our own transportation to games and practice. And mom never missed an opportunity to remind us that we could use our own "fat little legs" to get around.

In spite of this barbaric attitude, we played football, basketball, baseball, swam and even delivered newspapers at 4:30 a.m. We hoofed it to school and the Clinton or Beechwold theaters to see such classics as "The Night of the Living Dead" and "Hercules Unchained."

Looking back, I suspect she didn't shuttle us around to leave enough time housekeeping and to foster in us a strong sense of independence.

I recall her telling my wife that we kids were "Raised with a healthy dose of good old-fashioned neglect."

We had our share of family squabbles, and mom was a reluctant disciplinarian. She once used a fly swatter to break up a fistfight between my older brother Doug and myself. It worked. We were stunned by laughter.

Yet, she could freeze us with an icy glare delivered with clenched teeth.

Sunday mass was a family excursion. Everyone was required to attend, except dad, who was not a Catholic. After mass, mom would mosey through the vestibule and parking lot, chatting with friends and glad handing as if she were running for office. She was later voted president of the parish women's club.

She drank in moderation, preferring Canadian blends – with ice, water and lime – to bourbon or sour mash. She never imbibed after dinner and two were her limit. For this a grandson dubbed her "Two-Drink Betty."

Words fail to describe the impact she had on the lives of those closest to her. She enriched us in the way she lived. We will miss her.

Nothing else needs to be said, except this:

She was my mother.

May 24, 2003

Facing untimely demise, boyhood has unlikely savior

Is boyhood under attack?

Once the stuff of colorful memories that inspired writers such as Mark Twain, James Thurber and Jean Shepherd, it now seems that boydom is going the way of paper boys.

Part of the reason I say this comes from reading the cover story of BusinessWeek. "The New Gender Gap" catalogs the downward spiral of boyhood. I first learned of the article from Washington Post columnist Richard Cohen. His account led me to the story, which I recommend to mothers, fathers, grandparents, teachers and anyone else interested in the fate of the next generation.

The larger part of my interest in this topic is personal. As the father of two boys, ages 17 and 12, I am always on the lookout for anything that puts my experience in perspective or sheds light on their world.

The article paints a picture of a vexing problem which experts agree exists but are unsure how the problem developed or what to do to correct it.

The results of this educational/societal lapse makes it seem as if boys are a species unto themselves. Boys are more likely to drop out of high school, get arrested, and kill themselves or someone else. They are also more likely to be diagnosed as learning disabled. Across the country, roughly 70 percent of students in learning disabled programs are boys. The figure in the Sarasota school district is 69 percent.

Those who don't attend college earn less money, thereby contributing less in taxes. For dropouts the picture is bleaker. Studies have shown that dropouts require $40,000 in government aid during a lifetime, resulting in a net loss to taxpayers.

Some experts fault the educational superstructure, which they say is skewed toward the skills that come naturally to girls. Girls are good listeners and are able to sit still for long periods of time. Boys, on the other hand, tend to be more aggressive and will fidget and squirm if required to stay in one place for more than a few minutes. Dose 'em with Ritalin and corral them in special classes!

Other experts assert that girls are simply getting their due after supposedly being overlooked by teachers who were giving preferential treatment to boys.

What kind of future awaits our sons? With jobs requiring testosterone-fueled muscle moving overseas, can they find fulfillment in lawn service or fixing cars?

Fear not my fellow knuckle-dragging Neanderthals.

Inoculated against this emerging phenomenon is what appears to be a sub-species of the male gender:

Nerds.

That's right, those geeks with the soda bottle glasses, pocket protectors and graphing calculators seem to be holding firm against the onslaught of the nail-polish-to-nails set.

More women have been enrolling in almost all college undergraduate fields than men. This trend held even in the most coveted postgraduate programs. For example, 51 percent of the students entering medical school in 2002 were women, and 49 percent of those entering laws school were women.

The exception is engineering – the field that attracts nerds like a Dungeons and Dragons tournament.

Nationwide, only 20 percent of those entering undergraduate engineering programs last fall were women. At the University of Florida, 21 percent were women. At the University at South Florida, the figure was 20 percent. Only 15.5 percent of those receiving engineering doctoral degrees nationwide in 1999-2000 were women.

So, you fathers out there might want to reconsider forcing your son to practice harder at football, baseball or some other sweat-inducing sport. Instead, introduce him to vector calculus. It will probably serve him better.

August 9, 2003

To the hospital staff: It's been great, but I don't want to see you again

Room 2 in the intensive care unit at Sarasota Memorial Hospital has a view of a new parking garage under construction. Further to the south is a scattering of shops and strip malls that line Tamiami Trail.

Tethered to equipment that monitored vital functions, I craned my neck to give me an occasional glimpse of the sky, which varied between azure and grey.

Those who could see out the windows, however, assured me that the view was less than majestic.

But for most tenants of the hospital's ICU rooms, the fifth floor window view was irrelevant.

Victims of strokes, heart attacks or lingering illnesses, some left the ICU covered by a white sheet. For others, the next stop was a nursing home or rehabilitation facility.

And so it goes.

My visit to the ICU lasted ten days; longer than expected, but enough time to transition to breathing on a ventilator.

It also gave me a chance to get to know some of the
nurses and respiratory therapists who nudged me toward recovery.

Steve R. is a respiratory therapist who lives in Gulf Gate Woods. Although he has been a resident of Sarasota for better than a dozen years, he still speaks with a thick New England accent.

Blame his friends and relatives in his native Connectiticut. Every time he returns for a visit he reaquires his distinctive twang.

A touch of gray never looked as good as it does on Carol. A nurse, she grew up in Daytona Beach. Her close-cropped, curly black hair is highlighted by threads of silver that together resemble a tiara. It's not a product of age, she insists. She says she started getting gray at the ripe age of six. Yeah, right.

Her medical skills have earned her the acclaim of at least one physician, who credits her with diagnosing and saving the life of an unamed patient. In tribute, the physician sometimes bows gracefully when she enters a room.

A respiratory therapist on the night shift, Steve sports a barbed wire tatoo – a souvenier from a visit to Daytona during Bike Week – around his right bicep. Originally from Allentown, Pa., he's a fan of Penn State.

But it's a girl who has captured his heart. He gushes about his 2 1/2-year-old daughter. Steve and his wife are caring for a friend's dog. And the toddler has taken a shine to the canine. So Steve's promised her a puppy if she potty trains successfully.

Good thing she doesn't like horses.

Amy, a night shift nurse, lives in Orlando. She likes classic literature and is a fan of Paul McCartney. Of the ex-Beatle, she boasts that she once slept outside in the snow in Liverpool to meet him. It worked.

She's traveled to England several times pursuing McCartney, and once even talked to him at a coffee shop.

Cathy has two daughters, one a senior at Riverview High School and the other studying nursing at Florida State.

Her real name is Cathyjo, but only her mother calls her that.

Ken is a respiratory therapist originally from Long Island. He likes the Yankees and the Sunday New York Times. He has two daughters – one a Gator, the other a Seminole. The family schism makes for an interesting football season, during which he wisely remains neutral.

There were others, too. Louise, Scott, Jennifer, Charlene, Karen, Jo, Ed, Donna, Todd, and Judy from housekeeping, who dutifully tidied my room each morning while I feigned sleep. I hope I didn't miss anyone.

Thanks. Let's hope the next time we meet is at a party, or even a bar. I really don't want to go back to the ICU.

August 16, 2003

Struggle for home ventilator is a fight for life

Here's a riddle:
What looks like a water slide and sounds like Darth Vader on helium?

Me.

I've adjusted my vocal chords to the rhythmic pumping of the ventilator pushing air into my lungs, so I no longer sound like a Munchkin Land version of the infamous Star Wars villain. But, being tethered by a plastic tube to the ventilator, I can't escape feeling like an attraction at a water theme park.

Some of these changes brought on by life with a ventilator were expected.

Many of these adaptations have also proved to be onerous, especially for my wife who has accepted the role of primary caregiver.

"We're in a steep learning curve, " she is fond of telling friends and relatives.

We slid into this learning curve even before I entered the hospital for surgery. It was then we learned how few medical equipment companies provide respiratory ventilators for home use. Time and again we were told that most ventilator patients were in nursing homes or hospitals; home vent care simply wasn't an option.

One staff member at Sarasota Memorial Hospital said that he had never seen a patient go home on a ventilator in the six years he worked there. My doctors seemed equally perplexed by the lack of options for people who wished to live at home on ventilators.

Had it not been for a volunteer with the Lou Gehrig's Disease Association (LGDA), I might still be struggling to breathe without a ventilator, or still a patient in the Intensive Care Unit.

Pat Rager, a respiratory care practioner, sits on the association's Patient Care Committee. She was able to put us in touch with a medical supplier based in Naples, which provided the home ventilator and ancillary supplies and equipment. (In the interest of full disclosure, I should point out that I am a board member of LGDA.)

Throughout all of this, our health insurance company has behaved, well, like a health insurance company. Their primary goal seems to be containing costs. For example, they have rejected our request for a second ventilator, which will be mounted on my wheelchair and allow me to do the kinds of things other people do: shop, go to the movies, attend school and community functions, and church services.

We plan to appeal the insurance company's denial, and we'll probably succeed. In the meantime, I'm stuck inside with two boys, my wife, and the dog. This is a double-edged sword, since they are stuck with me. So, we could probably make a good case that the second ventilator would salvage what little sanity remains in the house.

There are some lessons to take away from all this. First, because of advances in technology, especially in the field of respiratory support, ALS and other neuromuscular diseases need not be terminal illnesses. Choosing life is a viable option.

In my case, the ventilator has improved the quality of my life. Breathing is no longer a struggle, so I have more energy and stamina. This comes at a price, of course. I'll be attached to this machine for the rest of my life. And my wife is investing much of her life to my care.

My wife and I have chosen this path. Together, we will see our sons grow up and find their own paths.

Secondly, perseverence and knowledge are perhaps the best weapons in dealing with recalcitrant insurance companies. Ditto for physicians and other medical caregivers. Establish your goals and don't be afraid to assert yourself. If your insurance company rejects a service, or refuses to pay for equipment, appeal.

It's your life, fight for it.

September 20, 2003

Mid-term's coming up -- time for a look at the cosmic report card

We're halfway through the first grading period of the new year, and we have a progress report for the 17-year-old to prove it.

For you child-free couples and retirees who waste your days and evenings playing golf and tennis, attending concerts, plays and movies and otherwise having a good time, progress reports tell parents how their children are performing in school.

I'd like to embarrass our oldest son by reporting his grades in English literature, calculus, biology and American government, but I won't. Consider it sufficient to say that he is performing well, given the gene pool from which he emerged.

Progress reports are excellent evaluative tools. They tell us in black-and-white, quantitative terms where the student stands at a point in time.

It occurs to me that all of us could benefit from such a tool. And I'm not talking about performance reviews at work.

They are useful for defining strengths and weaknesses for that part of life, but there is much more to life than work.

There are golf, tennis, fishing, baseball playoffs, college football, kids' soccer, eating, shopping, laundry, and cleaning the bathroom. How do we evaluate ourselves as individuals? By how much money we earn? How our stocks perform? Our golf handicap? How much we can bench press? The kind of car we drive? The size of our house?

For some, those are legitimate evaluative markers. Others might value more spiritual or emotional qualities. What is needed, then, is a progress report to evaluate those elements that define us. Establishing those factors requires deep reflection – give yourself at least five minutes.

For me, those elements are health; mobility; family, intellectual, spiritual and creative growth; television; and college football.

So tie me to the whipping post and get on with my public self-evaluation.

College football: This is the easiest for me, kind of like eating dessert first. My alma mater is 3-0 and ranked in the top five nationally. They've struggled on and off the field. Should be an interesting season. Grade: B+.

Television: We fired the cable company and opted for satellite. Where we once received 50 channels of garbage, we now get 150 for roughly the same price. Grade: C.

Health: Put bluntly, my health sucks. I use a ventilator to breathe and am totally dependent on others for dressing, bathing, and eating. Thanks to medical technology I am still here. Grade: D+.

Mobility: Closely related to health issues. An electric wheelchair affords limited mobility, but it needs to be modified to support a portable ventilator. Unfortunately, I am subject to the whims of knuckleheaded bureaucrats at Blue Cross-Blue Shield for this. Grade: D (Room for improvement.)

Intellectual, spiritual and creative growth: The key word here is growth. There is only one way to go, and that's up. Recently completed studies of St. Augustine, St. Thomas Aquinas, Aristotle and SpongeBob Squarepants.

Augustine's "Confessions," Thomas Aquinas' "Summa Theologiae," readings of Aristotle, and SpongeBob's technique for jellyfishing are required for well-rounded spiritual and intellectual growth. Grade: A-.

Family: With the exception of a short-tempered, thick-headed father, all family members – the mother, the 12-year-old and the 17-year-old – are pleasant and thriving. Grade: A- (Dad is hurting performance.)

Overall Grade: C. Humanity is a work in progress; and I'm no different.

There's plenty of room for improvement and growth. Need to focus on the positive characteristics of family members, and guard against belief that I'm always right, even though I am.

November 22, 2003

No matter how much is taken away, you always have something left

Whack the walls. And the doors. And the bookshelves.

Navigating the hallways and rooms of the house has never been easy in my wheelchair.

Maneuvering became more difficult a couple of months ago with the added girth of a ventilator tray and 40-pound ventilator. Riding behind the chair, the vent and tray sway like a concrete block on a swing.

Driving with this added girth has been a learning experience. I found myself scraping drywall and wood where I once pivoted and glided past sleeping dogs and lounging teenagers.

It became increasingly obvious that something had to give:

The walls. The doors. And the bookshelves.

So last week, as my wife started preparing for the Thanksgiving invasion of guests and family, my health aide and I began the purge.

A set of bookshelves in the master bedroom was the first and easiest target.

Over the fussing objections of my wife, the shelves were emptied of their bric-a-brac, books and ceramics, which will become merchandise for a garage sale, to be held at a date yet to be determined.

This task consumed several hours, engaging all the family members: my wife, our 17-year-old son and his 12-year-old brother, and me. I offered directions from my wheelchair.

A couple of weeks later we were visited by a vocational rehabilitation engineer. His task was to evaluate my home-work environment for modifications and improvements.

He immediately identified two doorways to be widened and a wall to be removed to accommodate the wheelchair.

To me, these appeared to be insurmountable obstacles. Knocking down walls and cutting wider doorways were beyond my remodeling experience and ability.

Yet, the engineer saw quickly what needed to be done, and just as quickly he offered straightforward and simple solutions.

What impressed me was not just what he thought, but how he thought. If walls and doorways were a problem, then move, or remove, the problem.

Most of us are familiar with this method of thinking. We may change the values used in the evaluation, but the process remains constant.

For example, when the family appraised the items on the bookshelves a few days earlier, we applied sentimental values to decide which items to treasure and which were destined for the garage sale. This process of assessing and culling applies not just to material problems but ideas, virtues, doctrines and opinions as well.

There is not much positive that can be said about living with a degenerative disease. But since my ALS was diagnosed eight years ago, I've applied this assessing and culling method each time the disease has taken from me something I valued.

When I could no longer walk, I placed higher value on remaining mobile, but in a wheelchair. When I could no longer type and edit reporters' stories, I turned to voice-recognition software and focused on writing.

When I required too much care to work in the newsroom, my supervisors helped me set up a home office so I could write and contribute to the newspaper.

Unable to breathe on my own, I'm grateful for the technology that keeps me alive and able to interact with family, friends and coworkers.

With ALS culling my physical abilities, I have renewed my interest in reading Aristotle, St. Augustine, Thomas Aquinas, Locke, Mill and others whose ideas have endured and influenced civilization.

I don't mean to paint a Pollyanna-ish picture. I experience periods of despair and anger, but try not to let them distract me from life's purpose.

After all, there are walls to knock down, doorways to widen and a garage sale to get ready for.

February 28, 2004

Like this artist's renderings, life doesn't always paint inside the lines

Roger Skelton remembers nothing of the traffic accident that changed his life.

It was Feb. 28, 1980, and Skelton, the vice president of a solar heating company, was driving home from a trade show.

At roughly 2:30 a.m. his 1974 BMW hummed along a rural, two-lane stretch of SW 232nd St. near Redlands.

His next recollection is 10 days later, drifting in and out of consciousness in a hospital bed.

A car coming from the opposite direction had crossed the center line and struck Skelton head-on, according to published accounts that cited a Dade County Sheriff's Office report.

Whatever twists of fate brought the two drivers together evaporated amid the torn metal and shattered glass of that cool morning 24 years ago today.

The driver of the other car, William Harrison Mowell, was released from the hospital later that day.

Suffering from a brain stem contusion, Skelton spent the next 10 days in a coma. When he awoke he was unable to walk, had difficulty speaking and could not remember why he was in the hospital.

Then 29, Skelton had graduated from the University of Miami with a degree in philosophy and was pursuing an MBA at Florida International University, He was also holding down a full-time job.

"I was driven to succeed," said Skelton.

But the accident changed all that. Unable to care for himself, Skelton moved into his parents' home in Nokomis to reassemble the pieces of his life. Through therapy and rehabilitation he learned again how to walk, and renewed an earlier interest in painting.

His paintings are displayed in local galleries and studios. Beginning Monday, his work can be seen through March on the second floor of the Caldwell Trust Company, 201 Center Road in Venice.

Skelton also teaches watercolor at the Ringling School of Art and Design and is a substitute art teacher for Sarasota public schools.

If Mowell learned anything from that 1980 accident, it's not demonstrated in state records.

Before the accident that injured Skelton, Mowell, then living in Lake Worth, was arrested in 1973 for disturbing the peace and in 1975 for possession of marijuana.

Between 1982 and 2002, Mowell was arrested four times for driving under the influence and recorded two more traffic accidents, one resulting in injuries.

Now living in Lakeland, he was sentenced on July 29, 2002, for a DUI. He got a month and a day in jail and one year of probation. Mowell did not return a phone call for comment.

Skelton admits that he is sometimes frustrated by his physical limitations, but he doesn't express regrets about his life today.

Unable to drive, he tools around Nokomis on an adult tricycle that's customized with an extended front fork to resemble a Harley-Davidson chopper and festooned with an American flag waving over the back.

He rides the bus on his commutes to Sarasota, chaining his trike to a post near the bus stop at Laurel Road and Tamiami Trail.

He has an unsteady gait, shaking hands and slurred speech. It would be easy to underestimate his intelligence. Yet except for occasional short-term memory lapses, his cognitive abilities are intact.

Being pre-judged doesn't bother him, even when he teaches middle-school students, whose gossip and barbs can be especially cruel.

"I am what I am," Skelton says. "Life is too short to worry about what other people think." Without being evangelical, he says his work is a reflection of the Creator and he is merely a conduit. Still, he admits to a penchant for Scotch. "It doesn't even have to be good Scotch," he said.

The transition from a hospital bed to rehabilitation to artist has not been easy or smooth.

For years after his return to Sarasota in May 1980, Skelton was angry and disillusioned, frequently lashing out at family and friends.

But the accident, while tragic, created a bridge to a new life. Skelton's art reflects his journey from the brink of death and from despair to acceptance. There is no separating the art from the artist.

His work exudes soulful optimism. Experience seems to have inoculated him from the brooding cynicism and cloying commercialism that have infected so much of our culture: the spiteful lyrics of rap, the vacuous redundancy of sit-coms, and the sweaty greed of professional sports.

Sharp lines and distinctive features are replaced by splashes of color that form shapes and contours not always recognizable. Skelton is unapologetic for what he calls a "child-like quality and perspective" in his work. He knows that his shaky hands are responsible for it.

Did Roger Skelton's gift blossom because of the limitations resulting from that encounter 24 years ago, or in spite of them? We all have limitations, some more apparent than others, and we all are products of our experience.

Yet Skelton and others touched by fate's dark hand understand that contrasts give meaning to life. There is no hope without despair, no joy without anger, and no light or color without darkness.

Like Skelton's renderings, life does not always stay inside the lines.

April 24, 2004

Buttering corn on the cob and living life can both offer challenges

How do you butter your corn?

Buttering an ear of corn on the cob is not a simple task. Television commercials make it look easy. Just place a pat of butter or margarine on a hot ear of corn, and voila, the ear is ready for consumption.

As any experienced corn-on-the-cobber can attest, this method is doomed to fail. As butter is wont to do when it comes into contact with something hot, it will melt. The result is that the butter slides off the cob, and only a few kernels have been buttered.

For much the same reason, a knife doesn't do much better. So the question is less a matter of etiquette and more one of efficacy: can you butter your corn?

There is a pretty simple way to butter hot corn-on-the-cob. And it won't cost any money, either. But, you'll have to read on.

In some ways, the problem of buttering corn is similar to many of the difficulties we face in life. Things that seem easy, or seem like they should be easy, are not.

This is especially true for people with disabilities. They've learned the hard way that good health is a gift, and not to be taken for granted.

For the able-bodied, walking up a flight of stairs, taking a shower, eating a pizza, or even reading a book require no more thought than drawing a breath.

Yet, for those in wheelchairs, or whose bodies are wracked with cerebral palsy, heart disease and cancer, or even those with learning disabilities, such tasks can be daunting.

Since being diagnosed with ALS eight years ago, I've become more sensitive to those with physical difficulties.

The latest of these challenges is my speech. After I lost the use of my hands, I used speech recognition software on my computer to write, and correspond with friends. My voice and diction were still clear enough to talk on the phone, tell jokes, give orders to my sons, and suggestions to my wife.

Over the last few months, though, my speech has become more difficult for those around me to understand. My speech is at its clearest in the morning, when I sound like Elmer Fudd on three martinis. Later in the day, I sound like a tipsy Elmer talking while holding his tongue with a pair of salad tongs.

The upshot is that my wife has to help me write.

Now, my wife is a busy person. She has a house to keep, meals to burn, laundry, an incorrigible dog, and two boys to keep in line. So, she doesn't have a lot of spare time to help me with my writing.

For me, speech is like trying to butter hot corn with a knife.

Enter the state Division of Vocational Rehabilitation. They've installed a new workstation in my home and upgraded my computer's speech recognition software. The goal is for me to be able to yell at my computer, just like everyone else, so that I can work independently.

As promised, here's how to butter corn on the cob:

Butter a piece of bread heavily. Holding it butter-side up in the palm of your hand, roll the corn around in the buttered bread. It's best to use a heel of the bread, since it's less likely to fall apart. No need to use more than one heel – you can share it – just keep re-applying butter as needed.

The heel is quite tasty once it's been rolled around half a dozen ears and soaked with butter. So draw straws to see who gets to eat the heel.

Now you know how to butter your corn.

If the new software doesn't work out, I'll be looking for a new way to butter my corn.

May 1, 2004

North Port Commission could learn something from Pope Stephen VII

It's doubtful that anyone watching the North Port City Commission proceedings Monday night even heard of Pope Formosus.

But the commission's attempts to collect more than $22,000 in liens from a deceased property owner was eerily reminiscent of the infamous Cadaver Synod in which the ninth century pontiff was tried and convicted post mortem.

Ultimately, the synod came back to haunt the pope who persecuted Formosus. History is seldom kind to those who task the departed.

Formosus became pope in 891 and died five years later. His successor, Pope Stephen VII, had issues with Formosus. Eight months after his death, Stephen ordered Formosus disinterred, carried into the courtroom, trussed in papal robes and propped in a chair.

Formosus was convicted of crimes against the church. As punishment, Stephen ordered that three fingers be chopped from the cadaver's right hand, the body dragged through the streets of Rome and thrown into the Tiber.

There are no transcripts from the Cadaver Synod, so it's not clear what Pope Stephen hoped to accomplish by convicting a corpse. Most historians agree that Stephen was a lunatic.

North Port city commissioners didn't go to such drastic lengths as the synod, but one wonders what they expected from Robert Seckula, who died in October 1997.

Seckula owned a house on Talbrook Road in North Port. In 2001, roughly four years after Seckula's death, city code enforcement officials cited the property for a hanging television antenna, said Raymond Miller, an attorney appointed to represent Seckula's estate.

Apparently the City Commission doesn't accept death as an excuse for failing to abide by North Port's rigorous property standards.

"It's not our purview to go out and find out if the owner is alive or dead," Commissioner Joseph Fink said.

"When a man owns a piece of property, whether the man dies or not, he is responsible for that property," said Commissioner Barbara Gross.

Miller said the fine for the broken antenna was only $25, but accumulated daily and is now $22,819.97, which is the amount of the liens the city placed on the property.

Appointed by a judge to oversee the disposition of Seckula's estate, Miller said the commission's response surprised him.

Miller figured his request to forgive the liens would have been granted as a routine matter. After all, it would have been difficult for Seckula to have the offending antenna repaired, given his state of death.

Miller said he is trying to locate Seckula's heirs. But that doesn't help him with the house. City officials want the liens paid before the house is sold. Just how that would happen is not clear. Formosus was a pope and couldn't mount much of a defense from beyond the grave. This doesn't bode well for Seckula, who by most accounts was a mere mortal.

Miller points out that Seckula's estate has no money unless the house is sold.

At Monday's meeting, Commissioner Gross said the poor condition of the house threatens the neighborhood's property values. Others expressed fear that giving in to Miller's request would signal to others that the city is not serious about code enforcement.

If that were the case, then wouldn't it be best to forgive the liens so the property can be sold? Is the commission genuinely concerned about setting a precedent? Are they worried that North Port property owners will start dropping dead to avoid paying code violations?

For historical context, it's worth noting that Pope Stephen VII, Formosus' persecutor, was deposed, imprisoned and strangled to death by those who were appalled by the macabre and bizarre Cadaver Synod.

Perhaps the commission will hold a seance at the next commission meeting to persuade Seckula's spirit to send a check.

I wonder what the postage would cost?

September 11, 2004

Small talk becomes a big thing when you're no longer able to do it

I'm no longer on speaking terms with my brother.

And things are pretty dicey with my wife, too.

It's no one's fault, either. Blame amyotrophic lateral sclerosis (ALS), also known as Lou Gehrig's disease.

Nine years ago this month I was diagnosed with ALS. And a year ago in July, I stopped breathing.

That's right. I haven't drawn a breath on my own since I was attached to a portable ventilator. I have room air pumped into my lungs through a plastic tube that connects the respirator to a stoma, which, in medical jargon is called a HITT, or hole in the throat.

The last nine years have seen lots of changes in my life, as well as the lives of my family.

I've been conscious of these changes, some of which have overtaken me incrementally. My speech is a good example of this.

A conversation last weekend with my older brother, who is half deaf, and a shopping excursion with my wife, who suffers from selective hearing loss, brought my communication problem into sharp focus.

Being unable to perform many of the tasks required of fatherhood, I sometimes ask others to act as my proxy. Noticing the dog in contented repose on the couch, I asked my brother to gently prod her from her satisfied slumber.

"Smack the dog," I implored.

He looked at me and smiled. He hadn't heard a word.

"Smack the dog," I said, raising the decibel level a notch.

This time he saw my lips move and walked to within shouting distance, which for him is about 2 feet.

"SMACK THE DOG," I yelled loud enough to be heard across the bay. Desperate, he called for a translator – my wife.

"I think he said Magna Carta," he said to my wife.

"Smack the dog," I repeated.

"No. I think it was Madagascar," said she.

While the two of them discussed how history and geography often intersect, the dog, perhaps growing weary of the noise, sauntered out of the room.

The following day, I was in the back of our van with my wife driving. As we turned into a parking lot, I spied a man leaving a store with my alma mater's logo on his T-shirt.

"Look at that guy's shirt," I said.

I'm pretty sure I didn't say what she thought I said. And I'm fairly certain I don't want to know.

"Fine," she hissed. "I'll find a parking place. You know, sometimes you are a real pain in the !#@," she said.

I wanted to dispute her characterization, but let it slide. After all, it's better to have someone think you're a pain than to open your mouth and remove any doubt.

My gradual loss of diction has made me appreciate the gift of speech and how we take it for granted.

There are those who disdain small talk, but as one who can no longer engage in it I can testify to its importance.

"How are you?" "That was some storm last night, wasn't it?" and other Lilliputian phrases often open the door to more important topics. And the phrase carries different meanings to different people. For example, saying, "How're you doing" to my son carries a different meaning than if spoken to a casual acquaintance.

It will probably be some time before I can no longer speak. When that happens, I plan to read Thomas Merton, who found sanctity in silence.

Until then, I plan to make myself understood, even to the point of being a pain in the !#@.

October 16, 2004

Sign of the times: Temperature drops, but air conditioner keeps running

With hand painted black lettering on a day-glow green background, the sign was difficult to miss. It was about the size of those ubiquitous real estate signs and occupied a swath of land between a white fence and the east side of Albee Farm Road.

But instead of "House For Sale," its message was "See You Thursday."

Parked in front of a neighborhood farm market, it was much more than a call to commerce.

It provided proof positive that fall had arrived.

Like other family run businesses that, I suspect, operate on a razor-thin margin of profitability, this market closes during the summer. Whether this is because there isn't enough local traffic to sustain it, fruits and vegetables are in short supply, or it's just too dang hot to work outside in the Florida heat, doesn't really matter.

The reopening of these seasonal businesses can only mean that cooler weather is near and that part-time residents will soon be arriving from the Frozen North.

The sign and its underlying meaning was enough to lift my spirits.

And I needed it.

Events earlier that morning put me in a foul mood. My trusty health aide had called in sick, so my wife had to miss a day of work to take care of me. Our 13-year-old son was not cooperating and seemed on the verge of mutiny. And I found myself grieving the death of Christopher Reeve, which hit me harder than expected.

The weather is what it is. But people view it differently.

One person might think 85 degrees is too hot, while another might think it's just right.

Such is the case for my wife and I.

She is a creature whose natural habitat seems to be an air-conditioned room with temperature hovering around 75 and humidity not exceeding 30 percent.

My comfort zone has a broader range. I can tolerate higher temperatures. So when she is away during the day, I turn the thermostat up to 80. Sometimes, I even turn off the air conditioner.

The warmer temperature never escapes her notice, leading me to suspect she has a thermometer implanted in her head that detects heat like an ant ferrets out a picnic. As soon as she walks in the door, she begins fanning herself as if she were a bonneted Southern Belle sipping sweet tea on a plantation porch.

Noticing the weather forecast predicted a spate of cooler weather, I pointed it out to my wife over breakfast earlier this week.

"Humphhh!" she said with more than a hint of skepticism.

Now, I confess to an ulterior motive for turning up the thermostat.

True, I like the scent of pine and orange blossoms carried on soft breezes through open windows. And I would gladly trade the rhythmic chirping of crickets and the song of mocking birds for the mechanical drone of an air conditioner.

But that thrifty Scotsman residing inside me likes finding other ways to spend the $100 or so a month we save on our electric bill.

My wife says I'm cheap. But I don't like forking over any more money to FP&L than I must.

I have to give her credit. She put up with the searing 75-degree temperature for one night.

Before turning in the next evening she was fanning her face.

"It's boiling in here. The thermostat says it's 83," she said. "Can I turn on the air?"

The decision wasn't difficult. Given the choice between an overheated, unhappy spouse and saving a few bucks, I relented.

Maybe we'll be able to turn off the air by New Years day. That should make FP&L happy.

November 20, 2004

Giving thanks: Mending fences, good neighbors and Harley Davidson

Thanksgiving is just over the river and through the woods, so this is as good a time as any to count our blessings.

To be sure, friends, family and loved ones top the list along with life and health. I have a couple additions to my list, made necessary by events that transpired earlier this week.

To wit:

The gate had seen better days.

Made of cypress, it held up well for better than a dozen years. It weathered storms, Florida's unrelenting sunshine and resisted infestations of various insects and other plagues.

But this season's hurricanes proved too much. The wind had ripped away a closing latch leaving the gate to swing wildly in the wind. Hurricane Jeanne unhinged the gate, leaving one end propped on the ground.

So the 13-year-old and my health aide were drafted to the task of replacing the gate.

Although I am confined to a wheelchair, I did just about everything possible to turn a simple two-hour task into an afternoon of wasted effort and mistakes.

None of this seemed to surprise the 13-year-old or the health aide. Being a fledgling teen, son number two's surliness gene has just kicked in. He operates under the belief that adults don't have a clue as to what they are doing.

For the most part, that assumption is correct. His mistake lies in thinking that he knows better than adults.

Having served ten years in the U.S. Army, first in artillery and then as a motor pool mechanic, the health aide understands that there is a right way to do things and there is the Army way.

Substitute my name for the Army and you can see my role in developing this SNAFU (Situation Normal All Fouled Up).

I instructed the aide to remove the old gate from its post and use its profile to measure and cut the new gate.

So when the aide placed the new gate on a pair of saw horses, I told him to position a toy scooter at his feet.

"Put that scooter in the way so you'll keep stumbling over it." I said. This was not difficult since the garage is full of kid clutter.

Around the same time, the 13-year-old returned from a mission to borrow a power saw. Being a father, I hate to see youth wasted. So, I asked him to replace a piece of the fence that

had split. To do this, he would need to fetch a cypress slat from a stack of lumber propped in the corner.

"Just reach behind, yank the slat and let those boards hit you on the head," I told him.

Unlike most of my requests, his compliance was almost immediate. Dispatched by gravity, a pressure treated 1x4 found its mark, striking the 13-year-old on the head with a report that sounded remarkably like wood on wood.

I unsuccessfully fought the urge to laugh.

"Not funny, Dad," said the 13-year-old while simultaneously rubbing the knot on his head and glowering at me.

Having sowed the seeds of incompetence, I rolled my wheelchair into the street to view my handiwork from a safe distance.

I would probably be there still, if not for a neighbor who was happening by on a Harley Davidson.

Watching the battle with the gate, the neighbor asked if he could help. My response was unintelligible, which he must have taken for a "#*!! yes."

"Let me get my tools," he said as he pulled his Harley into the driveway.

With the neighbor providing much needed experience, the new gate was swinging easily on its hinges after about an hour.

Which brings me to the additions to my Thanksgiving list.

I'm grateful for neighbors who always seem willing to pitch in and help.

And I'm thankful for Harley Davidson motorcycles. Without them, the neighbor would not have seen my need for assistance.

February 5, 2005

State of parenthood: Suffering from delusions

President Bush's State of the Union address Wednesday night provides a good example of how parents delude themselves about their children.

Talking about Social Security, the President said, "If you have a 5-year old, you're already concerned about how you'll pay for college tuition 13 years down the road. If you've got children in their 20's, as some of us do, the idea of Social Security collapsing does not seem like a small matter."

The future of Social Security is an important topic, but parents of 5-year olds have more immediate worries than college or retirement. When our sons were around that age, my wife and I were concerned about teaching them that peeing near the toilet wasn't good enough. We even considered painting a bull's eye in the bowl to improve their marksmanship.

As for "children" in their 20's: Our friends who have offspring that age are just trying to get them to move out of the house.

Did you ever wonder why the only people known to speak fondly of child-rearing are those whose parenting days are far behind them? Retirees and grandparents smirk knowingly as young mothers struggle to control their screaming 2-year-old in the grocery store. It's also why only the parents of infants gush when talking about their babies. Parental boasting about teenagers is rare.

And of course, we parents pity childless couples and retirees who waste their time on the theatre, eating at restaurants that serve food on plates, and playing golf or tennis.

Parents are seldom realistic and often downright delusional about their kids. They want to think that their kid gets bad grades because of boredom; this is easier than accepting that their product of the gene pool is just, well, not the sharpest tool in the shed.

Sometimes these delusions diminish with time. More often, though, they manifest themselves in different forms. Parents need to manufacture fresh delusions to meet new challenges as children age.

I'm a good example of this phenomenon.

When our oldest son, 18, moved away to college last fall, I believed that he would no longer need financial support for day-to-day living expenses.

After all, we were providing shelter (a dorm), food (prepaid meals with the university); we even bought for him a bicycle so he wouldn't have to trudge to classes on those unbearably temperate Florida mornings.

We figured that the money he saved from his summer job would be enough for laundry, toiletries and entertainment.

But that was gone by the end of his first semester.

The mystery of the evaporating cash deepened when he brought a half-ton of dirty clothes with him on his first visit home. We knew he wasn't spending his money at the coin-operated laundry.

We found answers during some casual conversations. Who knew that buying pizza four nights a week would cost so much?

I'm not much better with our 14-year old son.

I held onto my delusion that he would willingly give up watching television for days at a time and learn to love reading books.

But when he started singing commercial jingles and mindlessly babbling lines from TV sitcoms, I convinced my wife to take action.

For every minute he reads a book, he can watch TV for a corresponding amount of time.

So far, it's working. He plows through his book chapter by chapter and earns enough time to watch "CSI" and some cartoons.

By the time he wades through "War and Peace" he'll be ready for college. By then I'll have some new delusions.

March 19, 2005

Warning: Teen brain under construction may cause cleaning frenzy

The U.S. Supreme Court decided a couple of weeks ago that executing teenagers constituted a cruel and unusual punishment and was therefore illegal.

For millions of parents of adolescents, the court's ruling affirmed what has been suspected for generations: that teenagers are not playing with a full deck; that they are a few bricks shy of a load; that they are several bananas short of a bunch; that their cheese has slipped off their crackers.

In reaching its decision, the court heard testimony citing neurological studies that found teenage brains are not fully developed. Apparently, the parts of the brain that regulate higher functions such as risk assessment, turning off lights and picking up wet towels and dirty underwear are under construction and won't be finished until the age of 50.

This ruling will resonate in every American household where teens are trying to wheedle more money for allowance while citing diminished mental capacities as the reason for flunking algebra.

Teenage stupidity is no longer an excuse; it's the law. It's been codified into the annals of justice.

And what parents had thought was sneaky behavior may be attributed to teenagers' lack of brain power.

How else to explain such actions as running up huge long-distance phone bills; inviting boyfriends over for make-out sessions while babysitting; and even (gasp!) cleaning the house, which is what happened to me last week.

Fortunately, my wife was not home at the time. Had she been home – she worked Sunday, leaving the 14-year-old to watch over me – this would never have happened.

Not many teenagers are called upon to care for their fathers, and this is not the first time the 14-year-old has been pressed into service.

In the past, the 14-year-old could be counted on to perform within the behavioral parameters of his age group. That is, he would complain and moan about having to sit with me while his friends cavorted around the neighborhood, played video games, watched TV and did the things that teenagers do these days to have fun.

I should have suspected something was amiss when he parked me in my wheelchair before the television and tuned the TV to college basketball.

"Are we expecting company today?" he posed to me.

"I don't think so," was my response.

No sooner had I spoken then the phone rang. It was my sister calling to tell us that she would be visiting that afternoon.

"Don't go to any trouble," said she. "We'll just order pizza and visit."

She added that she would be bringing her husband and his 13-year-old granddaughter, who had escaped the frozen tundra of the Midwest for spring break.

The 14-year-old paused momentarily to pat himself on the back for his intuition, and then started to act on his insidious plot.

At that time, I wasn't sure what he was doing. I had my back turned to his activity and was unable to pivot the wheelchair to see what he was doing. It was only after he passed in front of me with the mop that his plot unfolded.

He had already scrubbed the bathroom, removed a bag full of debris from his room and made his bed. I heard him behind me rattling around in the kitchen.

I'm not sure what motivated him. It could have been a desire to impress the 13-year-old girl, or the fear of his mother throwing a cleaning fit to make the house ready for visitors.

Either way, my wife knew enough not to raise questions. But she was suspicious.

"Did aliens kidnap my son and replace him with a robot?" was her reaction.

Maybe it happened while my back was turned.

May 7, 2005

For fun or profit, mowing the lawn has its own reward

The toilet is stopped up, weeds are taking over the butterfly garden, the pool needs cleaning, and we're just about out of milk.

Yet, the 14-year-old overlooked these family foibles and attached a half-dozen brightly colored balloons to the mailbox.

Flapping gently in the breeze, the balloons attracted the attention of a neighbor who was strolling through the neighborhood.

She came to the door as we dined on pot roast and mashed potatoes.

"I saw the balloons," said Cindy. "Is it someone's birthday? Or did someone die?"

My wife laughed and answered that the balloons were there to herald a new arrival at our house: a riding lawn mower.

Now, most folks don't see the purchase of a spanking new lawn mower, with a 40-inch blade and 13.5 hp Briggs & Stratton engine as a reason to celebrate.

But then, they never had to cut a hilly lawn of St. Augustine grass using a 20-inch self-propelled lawn mower that pulls to the left.

With his 19-year-old brother away at college, many chores the two brothers once shared have fallen on the lanky shoulders of the 14-year-old.

Cutting the lawn is one such job.

In terms of the family, this falls under the good-news-bad-news category.

For my wife and me it's good news. We no longer have to suffer through long drawn out arguments and fights over which of our cherished offspring must cut the grass or trim the borders.

For the 14-year-old, it's bad news. My wife and I know who's to blame if the grass doesn't get cut.

Even using the old lawn mower, the 14-year-old offered only token resistance when pressed into yard duty.

That's not to say the job didn't tax him. Standing nearly 5-6 and weighing less than 100 pounds, he struggled against gravity, the grass and the old lawn mower.

In the damp grass, his feet would sometimes slip causing him to stumble on the hill, lose his grip and stall the mower. Other times, the mower acted as if it had a mind of its own and meandered into the street.

More than once I witnessed his battle from the air-conditioned perch in our living room.

Some kids might have surrendered when faced with such obstacles. After all, he wasn't getting paid. His only reward, if one could call it that, was that he would remain in his parents' good graces. We have never paid our sons allowance for household chores. My wife and I are of the mind that chores come with being part of a family.

Although he sometimes griped about having to work around the house, once he began a task he stayed with it until it was done.

And so it was with the yard.

On the evening after the new lawn mower was delivered, the 14-year-old decided to take it out for a test spin. My wife and I watched him as he tooled around the front yard.

"I'll be able to cut the lawn at night!" he shouted at us above the pocketa-pocketa-pocketa of the Briggs & Stratton.

"It has headlights," he said as he and the mower disappeared around the corner of the house.

His enthusiasm for the lawn mower will undoubtedly wane. But it hasn't yet. In the week we've owned the riding mower, the lawn has been cut twice. Ditto for a neighbor's yard that he's being paid to maintain while they're away for the summer.

So taken was he with the new arrival that his mother and I have been able to eek more chores out of him.

He plunged the toilet, weeded the garden, and cleaned the pool.

He even volunteered to go to the store for a gallon of milk. But we wouldn't let him take the lawn mower.

August 6, 2005

Aliens among us?
Back-to-school shopping
provides close encounter

I've never bought the idea that extraterrestrials are living among us.

Much of my skepticism toward little green men is largely because I've never seen one, unless you count Freddy the Frog Boy, a regular sideshow attraction at the Ohio State Fair.

Well, Freddy fit the little and green parts, but I don't think he was from another planet. If my memory serves me, Freddy was from Steubenville, a town in eastern Ohio's Rust Belt that smells nearly as bad as Jacksonville.

This past week, though, I spoke with an alien.

She was not green or even olive. And she didn't have any telltale markings, such as antennae or nodules protruding from her neck.

But there were subtle indications that neither she nor the two children with her were of this world.

My wife and I had been shopping for back-to-school clothing for our 19-year-old son.

As they were checking out, I parked my wheelchair near the exit. Experience has taught me that if I wait there I can collect some extra cash because people mistake me for a panhandler.

With two children in tow, a boy who looked to be about 11 and a girl perhaps 6 or 7, she ambushed me as I waited.

"Are you doing some back-to-school shopping?" she said.

Behind her, a well-dressed gentleman wearing a badly fitting toupee slipped through the exit. A few minutes earlier I had watched him fumble with a wad of cash as he maneuvered through the checkout.

"Is your wife with you?" she continued.

I nodded and glanced to where my wife and oldest son were liberating a couple of Franklins from her wallet.

It was her next remark that tipped me off.

"I always get wistful this time of year with the kids going back to school," she said.

Wistful? A true earth mother is relieved to have the kids back at school. I guess the alien's training manual didn't cover that little detail.

Her children also displayed aberrant behavior.

The boy appeared to be staring off into space. Unlike real earth boys, he did not have his face buried in a Game Boy.

And the girl was alert and precocious; she waited politely as her mother talked.

Had they been real earth children, the boy would have been whining for something he didn't need and the girl would have been making her brother miserable. She should have been in his face, pestering and complaining.

They maintained their cover, and the three left the store as my wife and son retrieved me.

The alien training manual was probably thin on the behavior of earth children. Nor was it likely to say anything about sibling rivalry, which can be healthy but later blossoms into an ugly phenomenon called the FONE – Fight Over Nearly Everything - syndrome.

The 19-year-old and his 14-year-old brother are excellent examples of how FONE manifests itself.

Whose turn is it to do the dishes? Fight.

Green Day or Los Lonely Boys? Fight. MTV or Cartoon Network? Take out the trash or recycling? Coke or Pepsi, paper or plastic, coffee or tea? Fight, fight, fight, fight and neither.

Convinced that something was wrong with our happy household, my wife the social worker referred the boys to a family counselor. He assured her that such behavior is normal, and that stupidity is not a personality disorder.

There are times when the boys get along. Other people have told us about it. It never seems to happen when we are around.

In the interest of intergalactic relations, my wife and I would be glad to lend out our sons to help the aliens revise their training manual. Ten or 15 earth years should do it.

September 3, 2005

Praise for teen surprises parents

Son may learn to bring his school behavior home

My wife and I attended an open house at the 14-year-old's school. He's in the first year of high school, so Tuesday night we did our parental duty and met his teachers.

But shortly after hearing his teachers describe the 14-year-old, it became clear that something was wrong.

The experience made me wonder if they were talking about someone else's kid. The other possibility is some kind of weird hysterical dementia caused by spiking the water supply with LSD. But as no one else has reported any hallucinations – such as believing that Republicans want to save Social Security or that Democrats have an alternative – my suspicions seem warranted.

His teachers were using terms and phrases not usually associated with the 14-year-old.

"He's a hard worker," a couple of teachers remarked.

Obviously, they've never asked him to sweep the garage, scour the bathroom or wash the dishes.

Some other teachers said he was "pleasant."

Yeah, right. Try getting him to turn off his XBox and go to bed.

Still another educator said he wished all of his students were as "cooperative" as the 14-year-old.

My mind raced back to this past summer when my wife asked he and his 19-year-old brother to take the trash and recycling to the street. They argued for 45 minutes over a five-minute job.

I'm probably not the first parent to react with astonishment when others have words of praise for a son or daughter. Parenting experts say that kids often save their worst behavior for home. They do this because they feel safe acting out in front of their parents and siblings.

While it can be exasperating, such unruly behavior can be a sign of a healthy home life.

Eventually, behavior at home melds with the higher expectations outside the home. The result is often a pleasant and well-adjusted adult.

I consider myself somewhat of an authority when it comes to the different views of parents, teachers and kids. My expertise dates back a generation.

My mother would attend PTA meetings with my grade school teachers.

I recall her coming home with fresh dispatches of my progress and attitude toward school.

These reports were delivered through clenched teeth and an icy stare that was as welcome as a bucket of cold water on a Midwest winter day.

"You're not trying hard enough," she hissed. "You're not living up to your potential." These one-sided conversations invariably ended with Mom saying she was "sick of seeing C's" on my report card. "I'm getting C-sick," was her clever-but-not-funny double entendre.

Virtually all my teachers at Immaculate Conception grade school, from Sister Ralph in first grade to Sister Donna Marie in eighth grade, offered my mother the same report, which made me believe the Franciscan nuns had been discussing my academic shortcomings.

Eager to participate in his schooling, my wife would go to any length to meet with our oldest son's teachers.

I did not share my wife's enthusiasm for this element of parenting. I figured that being a college graduate had earned me a pass.

But after spending a few nights on the sofa, I saw the wisdom of my wife's point of view.

Far from the effusive praise heaped on his younger brother, though, the oldest son's teachers offered neutral evaluations.

"We're glad he's been able to wear matching socks," I remember his eighth-grade science teacher told us. That was the year we switched to buying only white socks.

This served to jade my perspective toward the value of parent-teacher meetings.

So the 14-year-old probably is hard-working, pleasant and cooperative. I'm looking forward to when he's like that at home.

November 19, 2005

Goodbye turkey; it's been great

Are you thankful? Of course you are.

But if you're like me, you've probably slipped into a routine and don't dwell much on the habits and virtues of daily living. That's as it should be.

If you go to church or synagogue, giving thanks is a significant part of the service. But for what are you thankful?

Health was probably high on the list, as were family and friends.

But was good fortune mentioned?

This time a year ago, many of our friends and neighbors in Punta Gorda and Port Charlotte were reeling from the effects of a devastating hurricane season.

We were spared this year. But as we all know, Katrina wreaked havoc in Mississippi and Louisiana. No doubt witnessing such pain and anguish brought many of us to mutter, "There but for the grace of God go I."

While those of us who live on the Gulf Coast have become accustomed to the gracious grin of good fortune, the difference between this year and last can be measured as the sum of knowledge gained: Now we know how lucky we are.

That said, this Thanksgiving could mark a sad milestone for me – it may be the last time I taste turkey, sweet potatoes, dressing, cranberry-orange sauce and all the other accoutrements of the Thanksgiving feast.

Thanksgiving holds so many memories; our collective remembrances form a cultural tapestry that gives us touchstones to the past.

But the unrelenting march of this disease could limit my ability to eat normally. I suffer from amyotrophic lateral sclerosis, commonly known as Lou Gehrig's disease, which is a progressive neuromuscular disease that affects motor skills but not intellectual functioning.

The inability to eat normally will be another payment, or another notch, as my wife and I refer to the disease's dues that must be indemnified.

Mealtime is becoming an obstacle for me. Swallowing is not yet a problem, but chewing requires so much energy I probably burn more calories chewing my food than the number I consume.

The answer for me is a feeding tube, also known as a PEG tube. PEG stands for percutaneous (through the skin) endoscopic gastrotomy (stomach tube).

My understanding is that the tube protrudes from my stomach much like a pressure valve on a car tire.

I probably won't have the PEG tube put in until next fall or summer. And I'm not wedded to this decision.

You all are probably getting misty thinking about all the wonderful foodstuffs I'll be missing. Oh, the boxes of macaroni and cheese! Oh, the succulent morsels of Mrs. Paul's fish sticks!

But to keep our spirits up, let me share some PEG tube lore I came across.

A man with stomach cancer was about to have a PEG tube installed, and his doctor told him he had to quit drinking. So, the PEG tube was implanted to his wife's specifications.

It was equipped with a pop-out valve – much like the meat thermometer embedded in turkeys that will be so golden brown and delicious come Thursday. When he imbibed, the alcohol in the booze would expand and the valve would pop out. That way she could tell when he drank and respond accordingly.

I guess the slurred speech and wobbly gait weren't enough to give him away!

Finally, this closing note:

Over the years of writing this column, I've received many warm-hearted e-mails and letters from readers.

I want to say "Thanks" to all those who have written, and also to those who've read this column. Happy Thanksgiving.

December 10, 2005

Christmas definitely a work in progress

G ot your shopping done yet? Are the decorations up? Cookies baked? Lights hung? Have you adjusted your attitude?

These activities should be near the top of any seasonal to-do list. They don't guarantee a happy holiday, but they sure help.

For me, the answers are: partly, yes; some are; no; they fell; don't own one; and working on it.

But we – the Trusty Health Aide and I – made some progress this week.

Since Thanksgiving, I've logged three excursions to the mall and two trips to a major discount department store. Thanksgiving is around the time the 14-year-old stowed away the Halloween decorations. And because he was climbing into the attic, he merrily fetched the tree, ornaments and lights.

Although no one has started making cookies yet, my wife said she will begin this week. It's safe to forecast an accumulation of fat cells around my midsection this holiday season.

The Trusty Health Aide spent the better part of a day hanging icicle lights around the back porch. But they fell in the raging fury of an evening shower.

As for my attitude, it may surprise some that I'm not blessed with a bubbly personality or sunny disposition. My attitude is a work in progress.

I confess to being an in-the-closet shopper. The popular cliche is that men don't like to shop. And up until 10 years ago, I would have liked to play golf, watch television, or contract poison ivy rather than trek to the mall.

But the past decade has seen many changes. In 1995 I was diagnosed with ALS. Now, I use a wheelchair to get around. Shopping malls, department stores and grocers are some of the more accessible places for wheelchairs.

So, I find myself looking forward to an occasional trip to the mall.

My wife still gets upset that retailers fill aisles with racks of merchandise that make it difficult for people in wheelchairs to maneuver. And she becomes angry with me if I refer to shopping as "bowling." Nor does she like it if I hit clerks and pedestrians or knock down displays with my wheelchair.

And the advent of online shopping has made trips to the mall a rare necessity.

So, I've been able to buy some items online and on sale, which has taken the frantic edge off buying gifts.

Perhaps most importantly, I've spent more time thinking about what to buy for those on my list rather than going from store to store searching for gift ideas. And even though I won't buy the 19-year-old a car or an ATV for his younger brother, it's the thought that counts, right?

Decorations? Well, we have the pre-lit Christmas tree up in the living room; and the pre-lit palm tree is in the family room. The 14-year-old hung the stockings over the fireplace and he put some ornaments on the tree.

There are many more decorations to hang both inside and outside. The 14-year-old will be hanging outdoor lights Sunday while I watch football on TV.

I haven't told my wife that she's going to make Christmas cookies while the 14-year-old is putting up lights. While he's on the roof he can clean out the gutters. I'll let my wife tell him that. Merry Christmas honey.

June 24, 2006

Refugees teach us valuable lesson

The photograph, and others like it, has been printed and reprinted so often that it has become a cliche.

A pair of large brown eyes stare back at the camera. The child is lying in a makeshift hospital. The camera has captured a pair of black flies dancing on the subject's face.

Stomach distended from lack of food and joints swollen with rickets, the caption tells us of the effort of doctors to save this one from death.

Is the child a boy or a girl? We aren't told. Human misery and suffering are genderless. Bangladesh, Somalia, Ethiopia, Biafra, Thailand, Sri Lanka, Pakistan and Darfur. Each year seems to bring a new crisis.

Tuesday was World Refugee Day, set aside by the United Nations to call attention to the plight of the millions fleeing their homes to escape war, earthquakes, floods, fires, droughts and just about every other disaster, natural or man-made.

While the paparazzi fawn over celebs such as Angelina Jolie and Bono, who are willing to do their part for humanity, for me the message of that photo and what it represents is more personal.

As much of a testament to human misery and suffering, the photo also demonstrates human courage, survival and perseverance, and is part of the intellectual engine that keeps me going.

Maybe you've wondered, as have I, what makes these people cling to life? They have no future beyond starvation. Chances are that child died shortly after the photo was taken.

Yet they persist.

And the millions of us whose biggest worry is whether to have white or red wine with dinner wonder why.

With their limited education are they the keepers of some life-sustaining secret that only those living in undeveloped countries possess?

Perhaps our pursuit of material possessions has obscured our vision, blinding us to the obvious.

For me, the lesson here isn't about guilt.

After all, we didn't choose to be born into the wealthiest nation on earth, nor did they choose to inherit a world of crushing poverty, disease and famine.

Neither can we excuse a callous attitude toward those who are less fortunate than we are. I find myself wondering, if that child were to find himself living in the West with an incurable disease, would he choose to die? Or would he put all the resources at his disposal toward extending life?

Each time I find myself wondering if I have the strength to tolerate another day of living on a ventilator; of being confined to a wheelchair; of have others feed, dress and bathe me; of using a computer and infrared switch to speak and write; I think about that young refugee and his unspoken commitment to living.

At least I have a choice.

December 23, 2006

Your kindness was not unnoticed

Life can become overwhelming at times, and we lose ourselves in the day-to-day routines.

Yet buried within these routines are acts of kindness that help define who we are and what is important.

Repeated day after day, it's these small acts of kindness that bind us together as a family, neighborhood, community and nation.

Taken individually, those acts – the smile, the kind word -- might not seem important. But they take a new dimension when seen as part of the whole.

Over the years, I've been on the receiving end of thousands of such acts.

Family, friends, neighbors and strangers have visited these kindnesses upon me. They probably think I didn't notice, but I did.

Maybe you held the door open at the pharmacy or grocery store. I would have said thanks, but you wouldn't have understood. Maybe you thought I didn't notice, but I did.

Were you the one who offered to hold packages for me while I fumbled for my wallet?

Maybe you thought I didn't notice, but I did.

Traffic was heavy that day. But you stopped to let me walk in front of your car. You could have ignored me and averted your gaze, as many drivers do.

I'm glad you didn't.

Maybe you thought I didn't notice, but I did.

Do you remember that day last summer? It was pouring rain. And you offered your umbrella to me even though you were soaked, too.

Little things connect us with family and friends, too. You sometimes stop your van on your way home to say hello or just chat. Maybe you sent me e-mails or letters to tell me you're thinking of me.

You may think that I don't notice these things, but I do.

Although I only visit the doctor's office a few times a year, I like the way he talks to me as if I'm his only patient. And I like the nurse's smile.

I notice the clumsy grace of my 15-year-old son and how he checks on the wheelchair when we're driving in the van. "Are you OK, Dad?" he asks.

And I see the way he does his chores when his mother asks, even though he whines when I ask him.

You may think I haven't noticed these things, but I have. The way my 20-year-old son touches me on the shoulder when he walks past and how he yells at the refs on TV when a call doesn't go his way, I've noticed.

I've noticed how my wife harmonizes with the radio and how she squints to read when she thinks no one is watching.

I like to think I'm unique for noticing these things, but I'm probably not.

January 27, 2007

It's good to be the bad guy, sometimes

Let's hear it for the rogues, villains and charlatans.

We all know that there are angels among us. Some we can see, while others are concealed to all but a few.

Mother Theresa was one, as was Pope John Paul II. Others may live across the street or down the road. They volunteer at churches, hospitals, schools and wherever there's a good cause that needs attention.

At the other end of the spectrum are those who are notorious in their own right. They drink too much, smoke and carry on, and know cops by their first names.

These people do more than keep our criminal justice system operating smoothly – they make us look good by contrast.

We're all under pressure, it seems, to not only live our lives as righteously as humanly possible but to set a good example for others.

There are also those whom we admire in secret because they seem to have so much fun.

At this, I confess, I have been negligent. That is to say, I haven't done a good job at being a bad example.

Let's blame this disease for that.

ALS has been my constant companion for more than 11 years. It's a condition that destroys the neurons that connect the brain with muscles. The result is gradual paralysis of those muscles. Those with this disease usually die within five years.

My health issues robbed me of a chance to build much of a proper legacy for my sons. For example, when I stopped driving roughly eight years ago, I had no moving violations. As it is, I can't even cuss, smoke, get falling down drunk or even leer at shapely women who are not my wife.

Doing anything while paralyzed in a wheelchair and hooked up to a portable ventilator is difficult; setting a bad example is nearly impossible. Acting on temptation is nearly impossible.

This sad truth dawned on me as I watched my wife struggle with one of several discipline issues presented by our sons, 20 and 16. They resented being called to task and pointed out what they suspected was one of her shortcomings.

At this I realized both the futility of trying to expect a reasonable response from unreasonable offspring and that I was not doing enough to absorb their barbs.

It also demonstrated that parents lead by example. This applies not only to big issues such as corporal punishment, but to daily issues such as table manners.

For me this means doing my part to supply enough of a contrast so that our sons see my wife for the wonderful person she is.

Hey, it's a tough job. But someone has to do it.

May 26, 2007

Embrace mortality, then live and grow

May is ALS Awareness Month.
Did you know that?

Well, I did. But only because I received an e-mail notice about it.

I'm aware of it, all right. I'm more aware of it than I'd like to be. Disease is like that, I guess.

Most people never give their health a second thought until something goes wrong.

Then comes an eruption of awareness, which usually lasts a couple of months. Eventually, this is replaced by what I call the "Now what?" stage.

At this critical juncture, there are four possible outcomes: the patient becomes worse, gets better, stays the same or croaks – a euphemism for kicking the bucket, buying the ranch and lots of phrases that mean the same thing. Life, defined by the act of respiration, has ceased.

I know I was like that.

Shortly after being diagnosed with amyotrophic lateral sclerosis, also known as Lou Gehrig's disease, roughly 12 years ago, I became an encyclopedia of knowledge about it. Nothing about what I learned was hopeful.

This is what I found out: ALS is a relatively rare disease. At any one time 30,000 people have it, with about 5,000 new cases each year. Roughly 80 percent of those people die within five years of being diagnosed.

There is no cure and no effective treatment; neither is there a known cause.

I wish I had never heard of ALS, just as many of you wish that you remained ignorant of Alzheimer's, heart disease, cerebral palsy, diabetes, Crohn's disease or any of the dozens of types of cancer.

Where would we be without war, disease, pestilence and famine?

Without the apocalyptic drumbeat of those horsemen urging us forward, humankind may never have birthed great ideas.

Michelangelo would never have painted the Sistine Chapel, Beethoven would not have composed his Fifth Symphony, we wouldn't have heard of Lincoln's *Gettysburg Address* or Thomas Aquinas' *Summa Theologica* or Hemingway's *The Sun Also Rises*.

I'm not the first to recognize our own mortality as a motivational tool.

In fact, that is one of the philosophical lynchpins espoused by Dr. Leon Kass, chairman of the President's Council on Bioethics and an ardent supporter of the president's policy limiting embryonic stem cell research.

What are we to do?

Embrace our mortality. It's part of what makes us great and reaching for the stars.

At the same time, we should keep extending ourselves – personally and as a nation. We don't seem to be in danger of living too long.

After all, ignorance is bliss.

July 14, 2007

The trendy side of proactive parenting

Last week he was a goober. Now he's a goober with dyed hair.

Over the weekend, and against my better judgment, the 16-year-old dyed his hair. Now, I am faced with a dilemma: how would I look with black hair?

This goes beyond the question that seems linked to gender identity – 'Does she or doesn't she? Only her hairdresser knows for sure' – and is more about my parenting style and skills.

My parents dealt with teenage rebellion differently than I. They ignored it. They figured – correctly, as it turned out – that our friends, who were mostly like us, would influence us. These friends attended the same church and school as we did.

In fact, friendship formed the core of a network of support for kids. I suspect that is behind the continued success of the Roman Catholic school system, in spite of the church hierarchy's opposition to birth control and its 14th century views toward women.

Parents today are too busy to ignore their children. They prefer a proactive stance, which is why parents volunteer to coach soccer, football and Little League.

They figure that if anyone can abuse their kids, parents should do it.

I became a proactive parent by accident. It was a few years back, when body piercings were the rage.

At the time, I thought a nose ring, a tongue stud, or an earring would be cool. My wife was concerned about infection with a tongue stud, so that was ruled out.

Being married, a nose ring would be redundant. And editors aren't into redundancy.

A trip to the mall helped settle my quandary. There, a girl in a kiosk was giving away an earring with each piercing. She had bright blue hair and spoke with a thick lisp, which was probably caused by the tongue stud.

Arriving at home I was anxious to show off my newfound hipness to my sons.

I thought Wally and the Beave would be proud that their Dad had taken a giant step toward coolness.

Instead, I was vilified.

"Thanks, Dad," Wally intoned icily. "Now I can't get my ear pierced because you had yours done."

Then it struck me that if I can prevent my sons from tattoos, body piercings and other forms of mutilation, then why not?

So, while you pour your second cup of coffee, I'll be thinking about what color to dye my hair. I was considering something to match my eyes. How about bright blue?

July 28, 2007

A friend's acceptance of death is hard to take

Randy is gone.

He died July 11. He was 50.

Randy Rabold and I met when he signed up to play football in the Clintonville Boys Association league in the fall of 1970. He was 13.

I was an assistant coach and Randy was the quarterback.

Those days on the football field were not all we shared. We also had a disease in common. ALS killed Randy. Amyotrophic lateral sclerosis, the same disease that put me in a wheelchair and has me breathing through a ventilator, proved fatal to Randy.

We knew that death was near. This past winter, he sent me an e-mail apologizing for "wimping out" on his annual Sarasota visit.

Only a few days earlier my wife told me that Randy decided not to use a ventilator. Which meant that he probably wouldn't live through the summer.

Maybe there's enough of a skeptic lingering inside that I couldn't believe her, that somehow she was mistaken. Or that I didn't want to believe it.

I like to think that I sent him e-mails hoping to provoke a discourse on the value of life, and that Randy would agree, seeing how much his wife, Denise, and their three children love him.

So, I sent him an e-mail with an open question that he could answer deeply or not.

"Have you made a decision about venting?" was my question to him.

"We decided not to vent," came the reply.

No discussion. No revealing discourse about life and the meaning of death. Nada. Nothing. Zip. Zilch. Zero.

I knew then that Randy was lost to me. In many ways it was as if he questioned my decision to live on a vent. Have I done the right thing by choosing life?

More than 30 years passed without my seeing Randy, although there were snippets of information about him here and there. Which is how I learned that he had ALS. About three years ago, my wife took a call from Denise and arranged a lunch the next time they vacationed in Sarasota.

Time has a way of changing a person's looks and outlook. Yet when I saw him standing outside the Sarasota restaurant that day he had that same boyish grin that I had learned to trust when he was the quarterback for the West of the River North Raiders.

Knowing what a person thinks in the moments leading up to death is a mystery. Urged by my wife to send an e-mail to Randy, I declined. The only thought I had was to send him a poem by Dylan Thomas imploring Randy to "rage against the dying of the light. Do not go gentle into that good night."

Clearly not the message for a man who has accepted his own death. What did you expect from a football coach?

Printed in the United States
97689LV00001B/271-462/A